U0237151

Practical English for Neurosurgery Residency Training

神经外科住院医师规范化培训实用英语

名誉主编　凌　锋

主　审　徐安定　潘伟生

主　编　王向宇　[利比里亚] Augustine K. Ballah

人民卫生出版社
·北京·

Practical English for Neurosurgery Residency Training

Honorary Editor in Chief

Ling Feng（凌锋）MD, MS, Ph. D.
President of CBNS
Professor and Chief Surgeon
Department of Neurosurgery,
Xuanwu Hospital, China International Neuroscience Institute
Capital Medical University
Beijing, P. R. China

Editors in Chief

Wang Xiangyu（王向宇）MD, MS, Ph. D.
Professor and Chief Surgeon
Head of Neurosurgery Department,
First Affiliated Hospital
Clinical Faculty of Medicine, Jinan University
Guangzhou, P. R. China

Augustine K. Ballah BSc, MBBS/MD, MAIS
Specialist Neurosurgeon in Fellowship Training
Department of Neurosurgery, First Affiliated Hospital
Clinical Faculty of Medicine, Jinan University
Guangzhou, P. R. China

From:
Neurosurgical Unit
Jackson F. Doe Regional Referral Hospital
John F. Kennedy Medical Center
Ministry of Health
Monrovia, Liberia

Dr. Andin Xu

Professor and Chief Physician
Department of Neurology, The First Affiliated Hospital
Clinical Faculty of Medicine, Jinan University
Guangzhou, P. R. China

Dr. Wai Poon

Professor Emeritus in Neurosurgery
The Chinese University of Hong Kong
Hong Kong, P. R. China

Dr. Alvin Nah Doe

Neurosurgeon
Head, Neurosurgical Unit
Jackson F. Doe Regional Referral Hospital
John F. Kennedy Medical Center
Ministry of Health
Monrovia, Liberia

Peter Guy

Peter Guy English, Creating Positive Futures
Guangzhou, P. R. China

Dr. Isabella Opoku

Specialist Neurosurgeon in Fellowship Training
Department of Neurosurgery,
Xuanwu Hospital, China International Neuroscience Institute
Capital Medical University
Beijing, P. R. China

A User's Guide

Practical English for Neurosurgery Residency Training is a communication-focused course book. The book is useful for teachers of medical English and for medical practitioners who need to use English at work, either in their own country or abroad. It presents authentic scenarios between doctor and patient which allow for practicing conversations doctors are likely to have in a hospital environment. The book also introduces general medical vocabulary related to parts and functions of the body, medical and para-medical personnel, education and training, research and presentations.

With a workbook-based method it uses various interactive learning techniques to develop mastery of medical English and the ability to use and understand it in the health care setting. *Practical English for Neurosurgery Residency Training* for classroom instruction focuses on the language and communication skills that doctors require to make consultations more effective, using the five elements of good communication:

✓ Verbal communication

✓ Active listening

✓ Voice management

✓ Non-verbal communication

✓ Cultural awareness

The book teaches learners how to sensitively deal with various situations such as recording a patient history and assisting doctors in preparing for dealing with a variety of patients. Good practice demonstrates the impact of good communication on the doctor-patient relationship and enables students to become confident and effective practitioners in English.

Today, China is in a more open era. Not only can we travel, but increasingly, more overseas people are coming to China to access our medical services. Accurate communication with overseas patients in English must be a basic requirement for all medical practitioners with a moral intent to providing a quality service.

Due to the specificity of medicine and doctor training, our country is currently implementing standardized training for residents and specialists. Despite the prescribed and general English training, specialized medical English learning materials are absent from bridging general medical English and specialized medical English resources. Each 'specialty' demands its vocabulary and context, so Chinese medical specialists should become comfortable conversing with foreign patients in English using relevant terms and vocabulary while being sensitive to foreign culture.

This book is designed specifically for neurosurgical residents and specialists, providing vocabulary, phrases, body language and cross-cultural awareness in textbook form and simulated doctor-patient interactions. The book's content attends to specialist and general medical English, associated clinical cases, English explanations of medical equipment, and physical examinations protocols in English (including pronunciation), essential grammar tips, surgery explanations, medical documentation and scholarly communication. This book also pays attention to the cultural differences between Chinese and English expressions in medical treatment. We have designed this book to be conveniently used as a reference pocketbook for doctors of all levels.

As my mother tongue is Chinese, and English is my second language, I relied on several people to help compile and complete this English language medical handbook. Dr. Augustine K. Ballah grasped my vision for the Book, and as a result of his painstaking work has made this medical handbook a reality. Without his commitment, the book would not have resulted.

Thanks to Mr. Peter Guy, my old friend and my English tutor, for his careful revision of the original manuscript and Dr. Alvin Nah Doe from thousands of miles away for his specific revision and advice on the book's practical and accurate clinical aspects.

Thanks Professor Ling Feng for setting the direction required for publication and using the book in practical terms. Of course, I also want to thank my young students, whose desire was the driving force for me to utilize my spare time to write this book. I want to thank my colleagues in my hospital and department for their trust and help, which made it possible for me to do this work well.

Thanks to my family for supporting and understanding the need to sacrifice family time to write this book. Of course, I would also like to thank my readers in advance for uncovering information gaps and proposing amendments to develop the handbook into a pocketbook further that all doctors will cherish.

Wang Xiangyu, MD, MS, Ph. D.

Practical English for Neurosurgery Residency Training is for neurosurgical clinicians, residents, young fellows and beyond. This project began in 2019 in our quest to contribute to the medical English education of the People's Republic of China. Chinese researchers in the medical English education field have done tremendously well over the years; there is a high standard curriculum requirement and some available resources, like *The Residency English Manual For Chinese Health Professionals*, to meet the great worldwide awareness need to communicate in English.

My mentor, Professor Wang of the Department of Neurosurgery, First Affiliated Hospital of Jinan University, had asked me to review *The Residents' English Manual* used by the Chinese resident doctors in our hospital. As a first language English speaker, a medical doctor trained in China and one who understand Chinese medical Mandarin, it was easy to identify in our review so many direct Chinese translations, such as referring to a 'consultation room' as a 'checking room'; 'investigations' as 'inspections' to mention a few. This review led to writing a revised resource for practical English for neurosurgery residency training in our hospital; however, it is easily transferable to a medical English resource for all neurosurgery residency training.

The book focuses on common communication for doctors in a healthcare setting. Role-playing allows students the opportunity to practice the sort of conversations they will have with patients in the hospital. Emphasis is on understanding medical terminology and everyday language to facilitate explanations and instructions to be given to patients in English.

The book is divided into eight chapters covering the following topics: introduction to the human body, medical history taking, patient's examination, medical records writing, special medical documentation, case report writing, presentation at academic conference, and useful medical terminology.

Augustine K. Ballah, BSc MBBS/MD, MAIS

Acknowledgement

Thanks to Professor Wang Xiangyu for allowing me the opportunity to write this book. Every step of the process was under his calm leadership and support to inspire excellence in neurosurgery. Thanks to all the contributors, but special thanks go to Mr. Peter Guy for his careful revision of the original manuscript and cross-cultural contribution and Dr. Alvin Nah Doe, my mentor and Liberia first neurosurgeon, despite his tight schedule, was still able to review and advise on the practical and accurate clinical aspects of the book.

I want to thank the Government of the People's Republic of China, and it's China-Africa neurosurgical training program with the calm leadership and support of Professor Ling Feng for the opportunity to train in China, which set the path and provided the opportunity that led to the writing and publication of this book. Thanks to my China-Africa neurosurgical training program colleagues for their contributions and comments especially Dr. Isabella Opoku. This book was made possible from the practical experiences from teaching it to the young residents and fellows in preparation and by the generous support from my Chinese colleagues in the department of neurosurgery, First Affiliated Hospital of Jinan University.

Thanks to my darling wife, Sumon Boimah Ballah, my children (Augustine, Ausum Augustina and Mogata) for supporting and understanding the need to sacrifice the family time to be in China and contribute to the service of humanity.

Augustine K. Ballah, BSc MBBS/MD, MAIS

Contents

Chapter 1 Introduction to the Human Body

Chapter 2 Medical History Taking

Chapter 3　Examining the Patient (Physical Examination)

Chapter 4　Writing Medical Records

Chapter 5 Special Medical Documentations

Chapter 6 Writing Case Report

Chapter 7 Presentation at Academic Conference

Chapter 8 Useful Medical Terminology

Introduction to the Human Body

1.1 Information Box

Every career in health care begins with learning medical terminology. In this chapter, medical terminology for the body and their respective everyday term have been explored to help improve communication in the health care setting, especially for English second language health care professionals.

Medical terminology is a special vocabulary used by health care professionals for effective and accurate communication; one significant area of miscommunication is the incorrect pronunciation of medical terms by non-native English speakers.

It is vital as medical practitioners that you use terminology that the lay person can comprehend, in those situations where you have to utilise correct medical terms, pronounce them correctly.

For accurate pronunciation, phonetic pronunciations are provided in the text at every opportunity.

To assist you in correct pronunciation we have syllabized the terms discussed; this means, we have divided each word into the individual sounds that make up a word's pronunciation.

1.2 Medical Terminology of the body: Directional (Figure1.1)

No.	Medical terminology	Syllable	Everyday term
1	Anterior	an/te/rior	Front
2	Posterior	po/ste/rior	Back
3	Lateral	la/te/ral	Side
4	Right lateral Left lateral	right la/te/ral left la/te/ral	Right side Left side
5	Dorsal	dor/sal	Upper side
6	Ventral	ven/tral	On or near the belly
7	Medial	me/dial	Toward the midline
8	Proximal	pro/xi/mal	Nearer to
9	Distal	di/stal	Farther from

continued

No.	Medical terminology	Syllable	Everyday term
10	Superior	su/pe/rior	Above
11	Inferior	in/fe/rior	Below
12	Cephalic	ce/pha/lic	Toward the head
13	Caudal	cau/dal (cor/dal)	Toward the spine
14	Superficial (external)	su/per/fi/cial (super/fish/al)	Toward the surface
15	Deep (internal)	deep	Toward the center
16	Coronal plane	co/ro/nal plane	Frontal plane
17	Sagittal plane	sa/git/tal	Middle plane
18	Transverse plane	axial (axial)	Horizontal plane
19	Prone	prone (prown)	Face down
20	Supine	su/pine	Face up

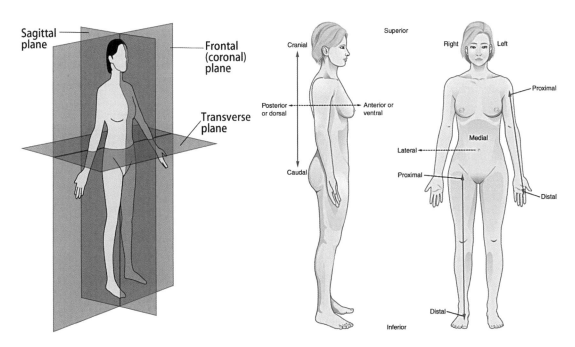

Figure 1.1 **Medical terminology of the body: directional**

1.2.1 Medical Terminology of the Body: Anterior (Front) View (Figure 1.2)

No.	Medical terminology	Phonetic pronunciation	Everyday term
1	Cephalic	ce/pha/lic (ce/fa/lic)	Head
2	Frontal	fron/tal	Forehead
3	Orbital	or/bi/tal	Eye
4	Oral	o/ral	Mouth
5	Nasal	na/sal	Nose
6	Buccal	buc/cal	Cheek
7	Maxilla	ma/xil/la (ma/zil/lea)	Upper jaw
8	Cervical	cer/vi/cal (sir/vi/cal)	Neck
9	Mentum	men/tum	Chin
10	Laryngeal prominence	la/ryn/geal (lary/rin/jeal) pro/mi/nence	Adam's apple
11	Axillary	a/xil/la/ry (a/zil/lea/ry)	Armpit
12	Clavicle	cla/vi/cle (cla/vi/cal)	Collar bone
13	Mammary	mam/ma/ry	Breast
14	Sternum	ster/num	Breast bone
15	Acromion	ac/ro/mion	Shoulder tip
16	Deltoid	del/toid	Shoulder
17	Abdomen	ab/do/men	Belly, tummy
18	Umbilical	um/bi/li/cal	Navel belly button
19	Brachial	bra/chial (bra/kial)	Arm
20	Antebrachial	an/te/bra/chial	Forearm
21	Thorax	tho/rax	Chest
22	Antecubital fossa	an/te/cu/bi/tal fos/sa	Crook of the elbow
23	Ulna	ul/na	Forearm
24	Carpal	car/pal	Wrist
25	Palmar	pal/mar	Palm
26	Iliac	i/liac	Flank
27	Digits/Phalanges	di/gits (di/jits) pha/lan/ges (fa/lan/jes)	Fingers
28	Genitalia	ge/ni/ta/lia	Genital
29	Femoral	fe/mo/ral	Thigh
30	Inguinal	in/gui/nal	Groin
31	Patella	pa/tel/la	Knee cap
32	Tibia	ti/bia	Shin

continued

No.	Medical terminology	Phonetic pronunciation	Everyday term
33	Tarsal	tar/sal	Ankle
34	Dorsum pedis	dor/sum pe/dis	Upper part of the foot
35	Phalanges	pha/lan/ges (fa/lan/jes)	Toes
36	Hallux	hal/lux	Big toe
37	Onycho	ony-cho (oni/ko)	Toe nail
38	Plantar	plan/tar	Sole of the foot
39	Metatarsal	me/ta/tar/sal	Ball of the foot
40	Calcaneus	cal/ca/neus	Heel

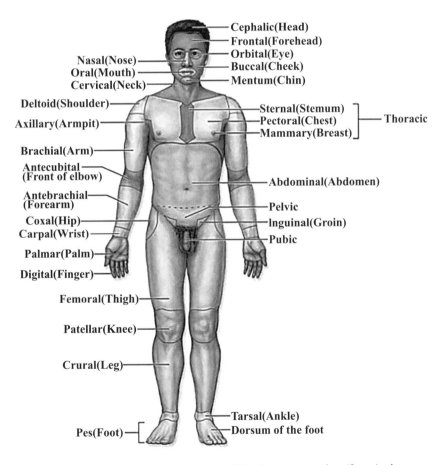

Figure 1.2 **Medical terminology of the body: anterior (front) view**

1.2.2 Medical Terminology of the Body: Posterior (Back) View (Figure 1.3)

No.	Medical terminology	Phonetic pronunciation	Everyday term
1	Parietal	pa/rie/tal	Crown of the head
2	Occipital	oc/ci/pi/tal	Back of the head
3	Nuchal	nu/chal	Nape of the neck
4	Thoracic region	tho/ra/cic (tho/ra/sic) re/gion (re/jon)	Upper back
5	Glenohumerus joint	gle/no/hu/me/rus	Shoulder joint
6	Scapula	sca/pu/la	Shoulder blade
7	Humerus	hu/me/rus	Upper arm
8	Olecranon	o/le/cra/non	Tip of the elbow
9	Vertebrae	ver/te/brae (ver/te/bray)	Spine
10	Lumbar region	lum/bar re/gion (re/jun)	Lower back
11	Os coxae	os co/xae (co/zae)	Hip bone
12	Iliac region	i/liac re/gion (re/jun)	Flank
13	Sacrum	sa/crum	Sacrum
14	Gluteal	glu/teal	Buttock

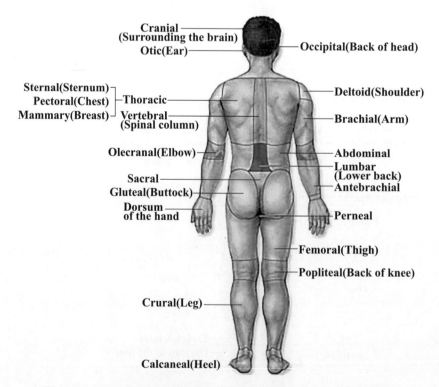

Figure 1.3 **Medical terminology of the body: posterior (back) view**

1.3 Grammar Tip: Collocations

English is a language of sounds; not just letter sounds as in the combination of /ph/. We do not say "*I bought a new p/hone*" but "*I bought a new fone*"…the /ph/ has an /f/ sound. The "sound" also applies to word groups. Word groupings follow no rules, they are combined just because they sound right. These word groupings are called "**collocations**". Some medical collocations are *tip of a nose , tip of the tongue , tip of the elbow , shoulder tip , corner of the eyes , back of the knee and inside the elbow.*

1.4 Cross-Cultural Awareness

Basic to understanding western medical culture is this: western patients only go to a hospital for one of three reasons, to have a baby, undergo surgery or because of a serious accident or spontaneous serious medical condition. Aside from the three conditions we just gave you, western patients first visit their family general practitioner (GP), normally located close to where they live (not in a hospital); should the GP be unable to treat the condition, they refer the patient to a specialist in that particular medical field. Again, the specialist will not be in a hospital (outpatient clinic) and will decide to treat the condition with medication or surgery; only for surgery will the patient stay in a hospital (get admitted).

In every interaction with a medical professional, the discussion and examination occur behind closed doors in strict privacy. The patient doctor privacy in Chinese hospitals is different from what foreigners expect. As a doctor treating a foreigner you must be aware and empathetic and accommodation to them.

1.5 Case Study

BR, a 70-year-old elderly woman, was hit by a bike while taking a walk near her home. The bike was moving at approximately 64km/h. As she fell, another cyclist collided with her, sending all three crashing to the ground. At the scene, BR complained of pain in her head, back, chest and legs. She also had numbness and tingling in her legs and feet. Other injuries included a cut on her face and right arm and obvious deformity to both her shoulder and knee. She had slight difficulty breathing. The paramedic did a rapid cephalocaudal assessment and immobilized BR's neck with a cervical collar. She was secured on a backboard and given oxygen.

After her bleeding was controlled and the paramedic immobilized her injured extremities, she was transported to the nearest emergency department.

The paramedic provided the prehospital report to the doctor in the emergency department. The report included the following information:

> Occipital and frontal head pain
> Laceration to the superior and inferior right ear
> Lumbar pain
> Bilateral thoracic pain on inspiration at the midclavicular line on the right and midaxillary line on the left.
> Dull aching pain of the posterior proximal right femoral
> Bilateral paresthesia of distal lower legs
> Posterior deformity of the left humerus

At the hospital, the emergency department physician ordered radiographs for BR.

Case study question:

You are the doctor in the emergency department, explain in clear and simple everyday English the prehospital report of BR.

Note: Use the below standard terms of the medical terminologies in the report.

No.	Medical terminology	Everyday term
1	Cephalocaudal	Head to toes
2	Cervical collar	Neck collar
3	Occipital	Back of the head
4	Frontal	Forehead
5	Superior	Above
6	Inferior	Below
7	Lumbar	Lower back
8	Thoracic	Chest
9	Midclavicular	Middle of the collar bone
10	Midaxillary	Middle of the armpit
11	Proximal	Nearer to
12	Distal	Farther from
13	Paresthesia	Numbness and tingling
14	Humerus	Upper arm
15	Femoral	Thigh

Medical History Taking

2.1 Information Box

Both clinical information and imaging findings are necessary to explain a patient's condition; because, sometimes there is a mismatch where the imaging does not explain the clinical presentation. One of the most daunting tasks confronting medical students as they first enter the wards is to master the art of case presentations. When a new patient is admitted to the hospital, it is the responsibility of the medical student and resident on call to obtain a good history and physical examination (H&P) and then to communicate this knowledge to the other members of the medical team. These skills are continually refined throughout a clinician's career as they see more patients.

The patient's medical history provides the framework for communication about the patient's care. It is the central aspect of medical consultation. The three aims are:

1. To detect abnormal symptoms that suggest a lesion
2. To localize the lesion
3. Identify potential pathogenic process

The most commonly used for the history and physical examination (H&P) format contains the following elements:

1. Chief complaints
2. History of Present Illness (HPI)
3. Past Medical History (PMHx)
4. Review of Systems (ROS)
5. Family History (FHx)
6. Social History (SHx)
7. Medications and Allergies
8. Physical Examination
9. Laboratory data
10. Assessment and Plan

Correctly taking a patient's medical history will avoid a communication barrier; especially for English second language health care professionals. This chapter discusses the elements of the history portion of the clinical information to be communicated to other medical team members, focusing on using correct medical terminology and simple terms.

2.2 Summary of Medical Terminology Versus Everyday Term in Recording Medical History

In English, medical terminology is not generally used in everyday language. Most patients will understand simple terms but may not understand medical terminology. Using medical terminology instead of everyday term when taking a patient's medical history, and explaining diseases or treatment to patients may be a communication barrier. A communication barrier is something that stops the easy flow of communication or information sharing between people.

Before you start, answer the following questions:

1. Do you try to use simple terms so patients can understand you?

2. Do you think doctors should use medical terms to reassure their patients about their professionalism?

3. Should patients be allowed to have the right to decide their treatment, or should their doctors make all the decisions?

No.	Medical terminology	Syllable	Everyday term
1	Loss of consciousness	con/scious/ness	Passed out
2	Cerebral hemorrhage	ce/re/bal (se/re/bal) he/mor/rhage (he/mor/ridge)	Bleeding in the brain
3	Vomiting	vo/mi/ting	Bringing up food
4	Indigestion	in/di/ge/s/tion (in/di/je/stion)	Stomach problem
5	Pain	pain	Unpleasant feeling
6	Deep vein thrombosis (DVT)	vein (vain) throm/bo/sis	Blood clot in one of the deep vein of the lower leg
7	Hypoglycemia	hy/po/gly/ce/mia (hy/po/gli/see/mea)	Abnormal low blood sugar
8	Malaise	ma/laise	Feeling queasy/Uneasiness
9	Contusion	con/tu/sion (con/tu/shun)	Bruise
10	Wound	wound (woond)	A Sore
11	Diarrhea	diar/rhea (diar/rear)	Running stomach/ Passing loose stool

continued

No.	Medical terminology	Syllable	Everyday term
12	Dysmenorrhea	dys/me/nor/rhea	Period pain/Menstrual pain
13	Conjunctivitis	con/junc/ti/vitis	Red eye
14	Allergic rhinitis	al/ler/gic rhi/ni/tis	Hay fever
15	Rhinorrhea	rhi/nor/rhea (rhi/nor/rear)	Runny nose
16	Dyspepsia	dys/pep/sia	Heart burn
17	Cystitis	cyst/i/tis	Bladder infection
18	Respiratory disease	res/pi/ra/to/ry di/sease	Breathing problems
19	Allergies	al/ler/gies	Sensitivities to medication or chemicals
20	Epilepsy	e/pi/lep/sy	Block–out or seizures
21	Asthma	as/thma (asma)	Wheezing
22	Urticaria	ur/ti/ca/ria	Itchiness
23	Nausea	nau/sea (nor/sear)	Sick feeling
24	Hyperglycemia /Diabetes	hy/per/gly/ce/mia (hy/per/gli/see/mea) dia/be/tes	High blood sugar
25	Pyrexia	py/re/xia (py/re/zia)	Fever
26	Bradycardia	bra/dy/car/dia	Slow Pulse
27	Tachycardia	ta/chy/car/dia (ta/key/car/dea)	Fast Pulse
28	Hypotension	hy/po/ten/sion	Low blood pressure
29	Hypertension	hy/per/ten/sion	High blood pressure
30	Thrombosis	throm/bo/sis	Blood clot

2.3 Introducing Yourself: Social Introduction Versus Professional Introduction

Before you start, answer the following questions:

1. When you first meet a patient, how do you introduce yourself?

    Example: Using your title or your first name only.

2. Is it important to explain your role at the hospital when you introduce yourself?

    Example: *I am the doctor on call today.*

There is a difference between introducing yourself in a social situation and introducing yourself in a professional environment.

2.3.1 Greeting in a Social Environment

Socially, it is common to introduce yourself and ask *"How are you?"* In a social setting, the questions *"How are you?"* don't need a response. It is a type of formal greeting.

For example:

Hello, I am Paul. How are you?

Response: *Hi, I am Mary.*

Hello, I am Paul. How are things?

Response: *Hello Paul, I am Mary. Nice to meet you.*

2.3.2 Greeting in a Professional Environment

When doctors introduce themselves professionally, they may combine several important factors in the introduction.

These are:

1. An introduction using their medical title.

2. An explanation of their role in the hospital.

3. A question to find out the reason for the conversation.

For example:

Good morning , my name is Dr. Su. I am the junior resident doctor on call today. How can I help you?

Hello, Mr. John. My name is Dr. Yi. I am one of the doctors on this ward. What seems to be the problem today?

Hello, Mr. John. My name is Prof. Wang. I am the director of the department of neurosurgery in this hospital. What brings you here today?

Doctors from native English speaking countries usually introduce themselves to patients as Doctor +family name.

Example:

Dr. Johnson

When speaking to young patients, doctors may use their first name instead of their family name to establish a friendly relationship with a child patient.

Example:

I am Dr. Paul.

In English-speaking countries, using a doctor + first name to address an adult patient may feel treated like a child and be quite insulted. **Read the dialogues between a doctor and an adult patient and determine which dialogue the doctor introduces himself professionally.**

Dialogue 1

Doctor: *Good morning, Mrs. Johnson. My name is Dr. Su. I am one of the doctors on call today.*

Patient: *Oh, good morning, doctor. Thank you for seeing me.*

Doctor: *What seems to be the problem today?*

Patient: *I have not been well for a few days. I have a very bad headache.*

Dialogue 2

Doctor: *Hello there, I am Dr. Paul.*

Patient: *Oh, hello.*

Doctor: *So, what is the problem?*

Patient: *Oh, well, I have a headache.*

2.4 Starting the Patient Interview: Asking Questions Used During a Patient Interview

Before you start, answer the following questions:

1. Where can you get information about the patient's complaint?

2. Why are closed questions useful when interviewing patients?

Example:

When did the pain start?

3. Is it a good thing for patients to search for their illness on the internet?

2.4.1 Types of Questions Which are Used During a Patient Interview

During a patient interview, open questions, closed questions, questions with options and summarizing questions are used to help get as much information as possible from patients.

Open Questions:

Open questions "open up" the conversation. They allow the speaker to start giving information about what is troubling them. The patient interview should start with an open question.

For example:

What can you tell me about your problem?

Closed Questions:

Closed questions are questions that ask for specific information from a patient. They usually get a reply like "Yes" or "No" .

For example:

Do you have any allergies?

Answer: *Yes.*

Questions with Options:

Questions with options give one or two possible answers. The question may clarify a previous answer if what the patient meant is not clear.

For example:

Patient: *I have got yellow fluid coming out of my wound.*

Doctor: *Do you mean fluid that is almost clear and doesn't smell or a thick, yellow discharge that smells bad?*

The doctor asked the question which offers two possibilities to check whether the patient is referring to normal haemoserous fluid or pus indicating an infection.

Summarizing Questions:

After listening to the patient, summarizing questions can ensure that the doctor feels confident that they have understood the patient correctly.

For example:

Doctor: *So, from what I understand, you have been losing weight and feeling sick for several weeks now. Is that right?*

2.4.2 Asking for Patient Details

Before you start, answer the following questions:

1. What information do you need to check during a patient's admission?

2. Why is it important to ask the patient for their full name and date of birth?

3. Why might the doctor ask a patient for the name and address of their GP in certain countries?

> **Review the following items:**
>
> *DOB:* Date of birth   *Gender:* Sex   *Nationality:* Country of origin
>
> *GP:* General practitioners
>
> *First Name:* Given name
>
> *Family name:* Surname, last name
>
> *NOK:* Next-of-kin
>
> *Mobile Phone:* Cell phone number
>
> *Patient's Confidentiality:* Keeping the patient details in a secure place so they cannot be
> seen by people who should not access the information
>
> *Patient's Admission:* The patient coming to the hospital for the first time
>
> *Patient's Discharge:* The patient leaving the hospital after treatment

2.4.3 Asking a Patient to Repeat Information Review These Phrases

> ➢ *Could you repeat your date of birth, please?*
> ➢ *I didn't catch your date of birth. Could you say it again?*
> ➢ *Can you please say that again?*
> ➢ *Can you tell me your phone number again?*

2.4.4 Asking a Patient Why They Have Come to Hospital Review These Phrases

> ➢ *What brings you here?*
> ➢ *What seems to be the problem?*
> ➢ *How can I help you?*

2.4.5 Patient Centered Interview Versus Doctor Centered Interview

- In a **patient centered interview**, patients explain why they have visited the doctor. They can talk uninterrupted and explain their symptoms as they experience them.
- In a **doctor centered interview**, doctors may diagnose their patient's condition after reading the patient's notes and only listen briefly to what the patient has to say and ask few questions.

2.4.6 Explaining Medical Terminology to Patients

Sometimes you may need to use a medical term and then explain the meaning to a patient. To explain medical terms, you will use an expression like:

➢ *What this means is that…*

➢ *(Medical term) means…*

➢ *(Medical term) is the same as …*

Examples: High blood sugar, Fever, High blood pressure.

Doctor: *Have you had* **hypertension**?

Patient: *Hmm, what is that?*

Doctor: *Have you ever had hypertension before? What this means is that have you had high blood pressure before?*

Patient: *Oh, no, I have not.*

Doctor: *Do you suffer from* **hyperglycemia**?

Patient: *What do you mean?*

Doctor: *Have you ever had high blood sugar before? Hyperglycemia means high blood sugar.*

Patient: *Oh, yes, I sometimes do.*

Doctor: *Have you had any* **pyrexia** *in the last week?*

Patient: *I am sorry; I don't understand what that means?*

Doctor: *I mean, have you had a fever? Pyrexia is the same as fever.*

Patient: *Oh, no, I have not.*

2.5 Grammar Tip: Prepositions

In the same way, cement holds bricks together in a wall, and grammar hold words together in English writing. Among the most important grammar (cementing) "words" are **prepositions**. There are roughly 150 commonly used prepositions; the word "preposition" actually means "*place before*"; this means that they generally, but not always, come in front of a noun or pronoun. Prepositions are meant to show the relationship or connection between a noun/pronoun and other words in a sentence.

The most widely used is the simple prepositions that deal with time and place:

Preposition	Time	Place
in	With months, years, seasons, and long periods of time: *The hospital was open in 2008.* With periods of time during the day: *The Professor will arrive in the morning.* The amount of time needed to do something: *The patient examination will be finished in 30 minutes.* When something will happen in the future: *The OR will be ready in one hour.*	With geographical places: *You should see a doctor in Guangzhou not in your poor mountain village.* Places that surround the subject: *Please wait in the ward.* With containers: *Place the biopsy in the container.*
on	With days of the week, and parts of days of the week: *The clinic is on this Monday morning.* With dates: *The neurosurgery is on November 28.* Special days: *The hospital will be open on National Day.*	With surfaces: *The scalpel is on the table.* Things that can be thought of as a line (roads, rivers etc.): *The ambulance is on Guangzhou Road now, it will be here soon.*
at	Clock times: *The surgery is at 10:00.* Specific times of the day: *We will check on the patient at lunchtime.* Refer to specific points of time: *The nurse is busy at the moment.*	With specific places: *Meet you at the pharmacy.* With addresses: *The patient lives at 286 Beijing Road.*

2.6 Cross-Cultural Awareness

Many things comprise a country's culture, for example, food, clothing, music, history and so on; one of the most important is language. Most Chinese medical professionals cannot use English correctly, or foreign patients cannot use Chinese correctly, which creates a great deal of miscommunication.

In the great majority of cases, it is the responsibility of the Chinese medico to at least have a level of English that allows for relatively efficient communication with their foreign patients. Learning a second language is never easy; however, the Chinese medical professionals can improve adequately with some planning and time allocation.

To aid in this, we have attached an English language study plan that you may find helpful; feel free to adjust the time and subjects as best fit you.

This English study plan is meant to help you allocate daily time to study a particular English skill. The more time you spend practicing English, the better; however, this plan works based on *15 to 30 minutes a day, no more than 30 minutes a day*. If you do not like the "Suggested" format, write in yours.

	Monday	**Tuesday**	**Wednesday**	**Thursday**	**Friday**	**Saturday**	**Sunday**
Suggested	Reading	Speaking	Listening	Speaking	Writing	Reading	Email
Own							

Discipline	Explanation
Reading	Select a topic that you are interested in and read it aloud. Remember: keep a note of challenging vocabulary ,write an example sentence.
Speaking	With a friend/colleague, agree on a topic before the meeting, then get together and discuss. When one of you is talking, the other is listening and noting down pronunciation and vocabulary challenges. This practice helps both speaking and listening.
Listening	Listen to an English song, movie, or TV show. When the resource has ended, summarize what you heard, then listen to it again. Try to listen to the English language Podcasts are a great resource. An excellent free online listening site.
Writing	Pick a subject (maybe what you read or listened too), then write a 200 plus word story about it. Write a "draft", check for correct use of articles, tense, singular/plural, prepositions, etc. Ask a friend that has better English than you to check it for you.

2.7 Case Study: Doctor and Patient Dialogue

Case Summary Ⅰ : Presentation of Medical History

A 40-year-old female presented to the outpatient department (OPD) with the chief complaint of severe headache for one hour. About one and a half months ago, the patient started experiencing headaches but didn't pay much attention, neither did she visit a doctor for the condition. One hour before the presentation, the headache got worse for which she decided to see a doctor. The headache is associated with neck pain and nausea but no vomiting, no loss of consciousness, no numbness or tingling, no visual or speech problem. No known past medical or surgical history. For family history, her brother died from cerebral hemorrhage nine years ago. She does not smoke cigarettes but occasionally drinks alcohol.

From the above medical history, the doctor has the impression of subarachnoid hemorrhage (SAH) will do a physical examination and order a CT scan to confirm the diagnosis. Follow the patient's interview below:

Dialogue

Doctor: *Good morning, Mrs. Johnson. My name is Dr. Su, I am one of the doctors on call today.*

Patient: *Oh, good morning, Dr. Su. Thank you for seeing me.*

Doctor: *What brings you to the hospital today?*

Patient: *Doctor, I have a severe headache. I feel like my head will explode.*

Doctor: *Oh wow, I am sorry to hear that! When did the headache start?*

Patient: *It started about one hour ago.*

Doctor: *What were you doing then?*

Patient: *I was on the toilet; I was pushing hard because I was constipated.*

Doctor: *Do you have any other unusual feelings, such as neck stiffness, nausea, or vomiting?*

Patient: *Yes, I have some neck pain and nausea but have not vomited.*

Doctor: *Ever vomit?*

Patient: *Not yet.*

Doctor: *Did you pass out?*

Patient: *No.*

Doctor: *Do you feel numbness or tingling on your face, arm or leg, especially just one side of your body?*

Patient: *No, I don't feel any of that.*

Doctor: *Do you have any trouble speaking or understanding other people's speech?*

Patient: *No.*

Doctor: *Do you have any changes in vision, such as loss of vision?*

Patient: *No, but when the headache occurred, I could not see for a while.*

Doctor: *Have you ever experienced this same situation before?*

Patient: *I have had headaches several times in the past several weeks, but not as bad. This symptom is the worst headache I ever had.*

Doctor: *When did you start having the headache?*

Patient: *About one and a half months ago.*

Doctor: *Did you go to see a doctor for that?*

Patient: *No, I thought I was catching a cold and didn't pay much attention.*

Doctor: *Do you have any other medical problems such as high blood pressure, heart disease, high cholesterol or other problem?*

Patient: *No, I am not aware of any medical problem. I hardly even take medications.*

Doctor: *Any medical problem that runs in your family?*

Patient: *My parents are healthy, but my little brother died from bleeding in the brain (cerebral hemorrhage). Is this disease genetic?*

Doctor: *I am not sure about that since I don't know the exact details of your brother's situation. Do you smoke?*

Patient: *No.*

Doctor: *What about alcohol?*

Patient: *I drink occasionally but not too much.*

Doctor: *Okay, good, I will do a quick physical examination if you don't mind. I also think you may need a CT scan to help confirm your diagnosis.*

Case Summary Ⅱ : Presentation of Medical History

60-year-old, a known hypertensive with average BP 160/110mmHg and diabetic with an average blood glucose of 7-8mmol/L. He is regularly on nifedipine 1 tablet daily and metformin 1 tablet each before a meal (twice a day). He presented to the outpatient department (OPD) with the chief complaint of suddenly passing out at 7 o'clock, a few hours before presentation. About a year ago, the patient started experiencing dizziness on three different occasions but without loss of consciousness. He didn't pay much attention, neither did he visit a doctor for the condition.

A few hours before the presentation, the patient had a sudden collapse while in the kitchen preparing breakfast and lost consciousness for about 10 minutes, after which he was rushed to the hospital by his wife. He reported no convulsion, headache, nausea, and visual or speech problems but has right-sided hemiparesis. His father is hypertensive, and his mother died from cerebral infarction. He smokes ten cigarettes a day and occasionally drinks alcohol.

Case study question:

Write a dialogue between the patient and a doctor detailing the full interview for the patient's medical history.

Note: Use simple and clear everyday terms and explain the medical term where it must be used.

Examining the Patient (Physical Examination)

3.1 Information Box

A detailed clinical and physical examination helps make the correct diagnosis. The medical history should suggest a differential diagnosis and help you to focus on your physical examination. For effective communication and accurate findings, health professionals must follow some general principles and be familiar with the right vocabulary. General principles of a physical examination are as follow:

1. Ensure privacy before examining the patient.

2. Explain to the patient the process of the examination and ask for consent.

3. Adequately expose the area to be examined but avoid embarrassing or chilling the patient.

4. Carry out your examination from the patient's right side.

5. Gently handle any painful areas.

6. Avoid exhausting the patient from prolonged examination, especially the sick or elderly.

7. Ask the medical or nursing staff for advice about chaperoning. Male health professionals should be chaperoned when examining young females.

8. Systematically record your examination findings.

9. Identify the patient's active problems and differential diagnosis.

10. Explain to the patient the findings from the examination and possible assessment and management plan.

This chapter familiarizes the health professional who has a non-English speaking background with vocabulary and terminologies necessary to communicate with a patient and other health professionals regarding anatomy, physiology, and disorders/diseases of the neurological system identified during the physical examination.

The ability to discuss the function of the neurological system is important in a wide variety of medical settings. This chapter will provide opportunities for familiarizing yourself with form and language, which will help facilitate your language and communication skills.

3.2 Medical Terminology Related to the Nervous System

No.	Medical terminology	Syllable	Meaning
1	Agoraphobia	a/go/ro/pho/bia (a/go/ro/fo/bia)	Fear of being in a public place
2	Aphasia	a/pha/sia (a/fa/sia)	Loss or defect in speech communication
3	Astrocytoma	a/stro/cy/to/ma (a/stro/sigh/to/ma)	A neuroglia *(neu/ro/glia)* tumor composed of astrocytes *(as/tro/cytes)*
4	Coprolalia	co/pro/la/lia	Compulsive use of obscene words
5	Corticospinal	cor/ti/co/spi/nal	Pertaining to the cerebral *(ce/re/bral)* cortex and spinal cord
6	Decerebrate	de/ce/re/brate (de/se/re/brate)	Having no cerebral function
7	Dementia	de/men/tia (de/men/sha)	Irreversible loss of intellectual function
8	Dyslexia	dys/le/xia	Difficulty in reading
9	Encephalitis	en/ce/pha/li/tis (en/se/fa/li/tis)	Inflammation *(in/fla/ma/tion)* of the brain
10	Encephalomalacia	en/ce/pha/lo/ma/la/cia (en/se/fa/lo/ma/la/seea)	Softening of brain tissue
11	Epilepsy	e/pi/lep/sy	A chronic disease involving periodic sudden bursts of electric activity from the brain resulting in seizure
12	Ganglionectomy	gan/glio/nec/tomy	Surgical removal of a ganglion
13	Glioma	glioma	A neuroglia tumor
14	Hallucination	hal/lus/in/ation	A false perception unrelated to reality or external stimulus
15	Hemiparesis	he/mi/pa/re/sis	Partial paralysis *(pa/ra/ly/sis)* of one side of the body
16	Hemiplegia	he/mi/ple/gia (he/mi/pl/jia)	Paralysis of one side of the body
17	Heterophasia	he/te/ro/pha/sia (he/te/ro/faysia)	Uttering words that are different from those intended

continued

No.	Medical terminology	Syllable	Meaning
18	Hydrocephalus	hy/dro/ce/pha/lus (hi/dro/se/fa/lus)	Increased accumulation of cerebrospinal *(ce/re/bro/spi/nal)* fluid (CSF) in or around the brain as a result of obstruction to flow
19	Insomnia	in/som/nia	Insufficient or non-restorative sleep despite ample opportunity to sleep
20	Intracerebellar	in/tra/ce/re/bel/la (in/tra/se/re/bel/la)	Within the cerebellum *(se/re/bel/lum)*
21	Medullary	me/dul/la/ry	Pertaining to the medulla *(me/dul/la)*
22	Megalomania	me/ga/lo/ma/nia	Exaggerated self-importance, delusion of grandeur
23	Meningioma	me/ni/giom/a (me/ni/gee/o/ma)	Tumor of the meninges
24	Meningitis	me/ni/gi/tis (me/ni/ji/tis)	Inflammation of the meninges
25	Meningocele	me/nin/go/cele (me/nin/go/seal)	Hernia of the meninges through the skull or spinal column
26	Myelodysplasia	mye/lo/dys/pla/sia	Abnormal development of the spinal cord
27	Narcolepsy	nar/co/lep/sy (nar/co/lep/see)	Condition marked by sudden episode of sleep
28	Narcosis	nar/co/sis	State of stupor
29	Neurilemoma/ Schwannoma	neu/ri/le/mo/ma schwan/no/ma (shwan/no/ma)	A tumor of the sheath of peripheral *(pe/rif/er/al)* nerve
30	Neurotoxic	neu/ro/tox/ic (new/ro/tox/ic)	Harmful or poisonous nerve or neuron tissue
31	Paralysis	pa/ra/ly/sis	Temporary or permanent loss of function
32	Parkinsonism	par/kin/son	A disorder originating in the basal ganglia and characterized by slow movement, tremor, rigidity, and masklike face

continued

No.	Medical terminology	Syllable	Meaning
33	Psychosomatic	psy/cho/so/ma/tic (sigh/co/so/ma/tic)	Pertaining to the mind and body (soma)
34	Radiculopathy	ra/di/cu/lo/pa/thy	Any disease of the spinal nerve root
35	Seizure	sei/zure	A sudden attack as in epilepsy
36	Shingles	shin/gles (shin/gels)	An acute viral infection that follows nerve pathways causing a small lesion on the skin
37	Somnolence	som/no/lence	Sleepiness
38	Supra-ventricular	su/pra-ven/tru/cu/lar	Above a ventricle
39	Tetraplegia/Quadriplegia	te/tra/ple/gia (te/tra/pla/jia) qua/dri/ple/gia (qu/dri/pla/jia)	Paralysis of all four limbs
40	Thalamotomy	tha/la/mo/to/my	Incision of the thalamus

3.3 General Physical Examination

The neurological examination is part of the general physical examination. Although the neurological examination is covered separately in the next section. In reality, the neurological and general physical examination should always be done concurrently and described as a single unit. The examination generally proceeds from head to toe and include the following sections:

1. General appearance
2. Vital sign (V/S): T-temperature, P-pulse, RR-respiratory rate, BP-blood pressure
3. SHEENT (skin, head, ears, eyes, nose and throat)
4. Neck
5. Back and spine
6. Lymph nodes
7. Breasts
8. Chest: a. lungs b. heart
9. Abdomen
10. Pelvic and genitalia

11. Extremities

12. Rectal

13. Neurological examination

3.4 Neurological Examination

Although there are some variations in assessment style among clinicians, we describe the neurological examination here in a fairly conventional format consisting of the following seven subdivisions:

1. Mental status

2. Meningeal irritation

3. Cranial nerves

4. Motor examination

5. Sensory examination

6. Reflexes

7. Coordination and gait

Outline of Neurological Examination:

3.4.1 Mental Status

1. **Level of alertness and orientation:**

   multiplied by 4 (person, place, time and purpose): What is your name? Where are you? About what time is it? Why are you here?

2. **Memory:**

   a. Recent memory

   b. Remote memory

3. **Language:**

   a. Fluency

   b. Comprehension

   c. Repetition

   d. Naming

4. **Check for overall knowledge base, attention, concentration and calculation:**

   serial 7s start with the number 100 and subtract seven serially.

5. **Thought processes:** delusional? paranoid? grandiose?

6. **Thought content:** realistic? delusion? paranoia? the idea of reference?

7. **Mood** (patient reports) **and affect** (patient transmit).

3.4.2 Meningeal Irritation

3.4.3 Check neck stiffness, Kernig's sign, and Brudzinski's sign

3.4.4 Cranial Nerves (CN)

1. Olfactory nerve (CN Ⅰ): olfaction (scents can be tested in each nostril).

2. Optic nerve (CN Ⅱ): funduscopy; visual fields to finger counting and visual acuity.

3. Oculomotor nerve (CN Ⅲ): pupillary response (swinging flashlight test) (& CN Ⅱ), eye movement (CN Ⅳ & Ⅵ).

4. Trochlear (CN Ⅳ), abducens (CN Ⅵ): eye movement (test eyes movement in all directions of gaze).

5. Trigeminal (CN Ⅴ): facial sensation in all three facial innervated regions, V1 (ophthalmic), V2 (maxillary), V3 (mandibular) and muscle of mastication (tested by clenching the jaw).

6. Facial nerve (CN Ⅶ): muscles of facial expression (ask the patient to demonstrate smile, frown, raise eyebrows),corneal reflex (& CN Ⅴ).

7. Vestibulocochlear (CN Ⅷ): hearing and vestibular sense (whisper or rub finger for sound detection), use Weber and Rinne test. Expect Weber to show that sound is heard symmetrically via a vibrating tuning fork held at the mid-forehead and Rinne to show that air conduction is symmetrically greater than bone conduction when the tuning fork is first held on the mastoid process behind the ear and place alongside the ear.

8. Glossopharyngeal (CN Ⅸ): palate elevation and gag reflex.

9. Vagus (CN Ⅹ): vocal belt movement, oculocardiac reflex and carotid reflex.

10. Accessory nerve (CN Ⅺ): sternocleidomastoid and trapezius muscles.

11. Hypoglossal nerve (CN Ⅻ): tongue muscles.

3.4.5 Motor Examination

1. **Muscle bulk:** muscle mass.

2. **Muscle tone:** maintenance of partial contraction of the muscle (hypertonia, hypotonia).

3. **Muscle strength:** it is often rated on a scale of 0 to 5 with 0 designating not even a flicker of voluntary movement. As follow: 0–complete paralysis; 1– a flicker of contraction only; 2–cannot resist gravity, but moves on the bed; 3–resists gravity, but cannot resist examiner; 4–resists gravity and examiner, but not normal; 5–normal power.

3.4.6 Sensory Examination

1. **Primary Sensation:**
   - ✓ **Light touch.**
   - ✓ **Pain** (sharp *vs*. dull), **temperature** (cool *vs*. warm): broken wooden swabs and cold tuning fork are usually used.
   - ✓ Vibration and proprioception.

2. **Cortical Sensation:**
   - ✓ Graphesthesia (palm writing).
   - ✓ Stereognosis (name object placed in hand with eyes closed).
   - ✓ Two-point discrimination (identify two similar distributions apart spatially over either side).
   - ✓ Double simultaneous stimulation (distinguish stimulation with one versus two stimuli) *Extinction: loss of stimulus on one side on double simultaneous stimulation.*

3.4.7 Reflexes

1. **Deep tender reflexes:** biceps reflex C_5/C_6, triceps reflex C_7, brachioradialis reflex C_6, patellar reflex L_4, and achilles tendon S_1.

2. **Superficial reflexes:**
   a. Abdominal cutaneous reflex
   b. Corneal reflex
   c. Gag reflex

d. Cremasteric reflex

e. Bulbocavernous reflex

f. Anal wink

3. **Pathological reflexes:**

a. Hoffman

b. Babinski

c. Patellar clonus

d. Ankle clonus

e. Chaddock

f. Oppenheim

3.4.8 Coordination and Gait

1. **Appendicular coordination**

a. Rapid alternating movements

b. Finger-nose-finger test

c. Heel-shin test

d. Overshoot

2. **Romberg test**

3. **Gait:** Ordinary gait, tandem gait, forced gait.

3.5 Special Signs and Other Tests

3.5.1 Primitive Reflexes

No.	Sign/Test	What to do	What you find
1	Snout reflex	Ask the patient to close his eyes. Tap his mouth gently with a patella hammer.	• No reaction: *normal.* • Puckering of lips: *positive snout reflex.*
2	Palmo-mental reflex	Scratch the palm of the patient's hand briskly across the center of the palm and look at the chin.	• No reaction: *normal.* • Contraction of a muscle on the same side of the chin: *positive Palmo-mental reflex.*
3	Grasp reflex	Place your fingers on the patient's palm and pull your hand away, asking the patient to let go of your hand.	• The patient can let go: *normal.* • Patient involuntarily grabs your hand: *positive grasp reflex.*

3.5.2 Superficial Reflexes

No.	Sign/Test	What to do	What you find
1	Cremasteric reflex	This reflex can be performed in men. The inner aspect of the upper thigh is stroked downward. The movement of the testicle in the scrotum is watched. Cremasteric contraction elevates the testicle on that side. • *Afferent*: femoral nerve L_1, L_2 • *Efferent*: L_1, L_2.	• Present: *normal*. • May occur with non-neurological local pathology or previous local surgery. • Lesion in reflex arc. • Pyramidal lesion above L_1.
2	Anal reflex	Lie the patient on his side with the knees flexed. Lightly stroke the anal margin with an orange stick.	Visible contraction of the external anal sphincter. If no contraction was seen, this indicated a lesion in this reflex arc. Most commonly, a cauda equina lesion.

3.5.3 Test for Meningeal Irritation

No.	Sign/Test	What to do	What you find
1	Neck stiffness	Not to be performed if there could be cervical instability, for example, following trauma or in patients with rheumatoid arthritis. The patient should be lying flat. **Place your hands behind the patient's head.** Gently rotate the head, moving the head as if the patient was indicating no. Feel the stiffness.	• Neck moves easily in both planes, with the chin easily reaching the chest on neck flexion: *normal*. • Neck rigid on movement: *neck stiffness*.
2	Kernig's sign	The patient is lying flat on the bed. Flex the leg at the hip with the knee flexed. Then try to extend the knee. Repeat on the other side.	• Knee straightens without difficulty: *normal*. • Resistance to knee straightening: Kernig's sign bilaterally indicates meningeal irritation; if unilateral, it may occur with radiculopathy (cf. straight leg raising).

continued

No.	Sign/Test	What to do	What you find
3	Brudzinski's sign	Gently lift the head off the bed. Feel the tone in the neck. Watch the legs for hip and knee flexion.	Hip and knee flexion in response to neck flexion: Brudzinski's sign.
4	Head jolt test	A newer sensitive (but not very specific) test for meningeal irritation. Ask the patient to turn their head horizontally at a frequency of two or three times a second.	• No effect: *normal*. • Worsening of baseline headache: *positive test*. • Positive test suggests meningeal irritation is possible. • Negative test makes meningeal irritation very unlikely.

3.5.4 Miscellaneous Tests

Tinel's test

1   Percussion of a nerve at the putative site of compression (usually using a tendon hammer). It is positive when paraesthesia is produced in the distribution of the nerve concerned. Commonly performed to test for median nerve compression at the wrist.

Lhermitte's phenomenon

2   Forward flexion of the neck produces a feeling of electric shock, usually running down the back. The patient may complain of this spontaneously, or you can test for it by flexing the neck. Occasionally, patients have the same feeling on extension (reverse Lhermitte's). **Lhermitte's phenomenon** indicates *cervical pathology,* usually demyelination. It occasionally occurs with cervical spondylotic myelopathy or cervical tumors.

Straight leg raising

3   Test for lumbosacral radicular entrapment. With the patient lying flat on the bed, lift the leg, holding the heel. Note angle attained and any difference between the two sides.
   • *Normal* > 90 degrees; less in older patients.
   • Limitation with pain in the back suggests *nerve root entrapment.*

Head impulse test

4   The vestibular ocular reflex (VOR) keeps the eyes stable when we move. Our vision jumps up and down like a homemade video (referred to as oscillopsia) if it is lacking. The main inputs to this reflex come from the vestibular system in the inner ear and proprioception from the neck muscles. The information is integrated into the brainstem and leads to eye movements to balance the effect of any movement. The head impulse test is used to examine fast VOR mediated by the lateral semicircular canal and looks at the ability of the eyes to remain stable with rapid movements. It is useful in patients with vertigo.

3.5.5 Grading Systems to Predict the Rate of Mortality in Cerebrovascular Diseases

1. WFNS grading system

The World Federation of Neurological Societies (WFNS) grading system uses the Glasgow coma scale (GCS) and the presence of focal neurological deficits to grade the clinical severity of subarachnoid hemorrhage.

Classification:

Grade 1: GCS 15, without motor deficit.

Grade 2: GCS 13-14, without deficit.

Grade 3: GCS 13-14, with focal deficit.

Grade 4: GCS 7-12, with or without deficit.

Grade 5: GCS < 7, with or without deficit.

2. Hunt-Hess scale

The Hunt-Hess scale is a graded scale used to predict the rate of mortality based on clinical features seen in a patient presenting with an aneurysmal hemorrhage.

Classification of Patients with intracranial aneurysms according to surgical risk:

Category	Criteria
Grade I	Asymptomatic, or minimal headache and slight nuchal rigidity
Grade II	Moderate to severe headache, nuchal rigidity, no neurological deficit other than cranial nerve palsy
Grade III	Drowsiness, confusion, or mild focal deficit
Grade IV	Stupor, moderate to severe hemiparesis, possibly early decerebrate rigidity and vegetative disburbances
Grade V	Deep coma, decerebrate rigidity, moribund appearance

3. Spetzler-Martin grading scale for arteriovenous malformation (AVM)

Lesion characteristic	Points
Size	
Small (< 3cm)	1
Medium (3-6cm)	2
Large (> 6cm)	3

continued

Lesion characteristic	Points
Location	
No- eloquent	0
Eloquent	1
Veins	
Superficial	0
Deep	1

The scale is used to decide treatment risks while considering the anatomical characteristics of a cerebral arteriovenous malformation. The grade is the sum of points assigned to the size of the lesion, the locatwion (in or not in the eloquent cortex), and the presence or absence of deep venous drainage.

4. Karnofsky Performance scale (KPS)

Progression	Score	Description
Mild	100	Normal, no complaints; no evidence of disease
Able to carry on normal activity and to work; no special care needed	90	Able to carry on normal activity; minor signs or symptoms of disease
	80	Normal activity with effort; some signs or symptoms of disease
Moderate	70	Care for self; unable to carry on normal activity or do active work
Unable to work; able to live at home and care for most personal needs; the varying	60	Requires occasional assistance and frequent medical care
amount of assistance needed	50	Requires considerable assistance and frequent medical care
	40	Disabled; requires special care and assistance
Severe	30	Severely disabled; hospital admission is indicated; death not imminent
Unable to care for self; requires the equivalent of institutional or hospital care; disease	20	Very sick; hospital admission necessary; active supportive treatment necessary
may be progressing rapidly	10	Moribund; fatal processes progressing rapidly
	0	Death

5. Fisher scale

Description of Fisher Grading Scale

Grade	Description
Fisher I	No blood detected
Fisher II	Diffuse deposition of a thin layer with all vertical layers of blood (interhemispheric fissure, insular cistern, ambient cistern) < 1mm thick
Fisher III	Localized clots and vertical layers of blood ≥ 1mm in thickness
Fisher IV	Diffuse or no subarachnoid blood, but with intracerebral or intraventricular clots

6. Suzuki classification

Suzuki stage	Angiographic finding
I	Narrowing of carotid arteries
II	The initial appearance of moyamoya vessels
III	Intensification of moyamoya vessels
IV	Minimization of moyamoya vessels
V	Reduction of moyamoya vessels
VI	The disappearance of moyamoya vessels

3.6 Grammar Tip: Articles

Three of the smallest words in English are among the most important for clear communication; these three are called the ***articles*** and are: ***a, an, the***. These three words are often misused by English language second speakers. *"A"* and *"an"* can only be used with singular (one only) nouns and must be used in front of every singular noun or adjective in front of every noun when you first use that noun or adjective in front of a noun.

I will see a new patient; she was brought in an ambulance a few minutes ago.

"...a new patient..." means that the doctor will see one of many new patients. *"...in an ambulance..."* means the patient was brought to the hospital in any one of many ambulances. "A" and "an" are referred to as the ***indefinite articles*** because they can refer to any one of many of the same thing. Notice in the example above, "an" in front of a noun starting with a vowel *(a,e, i,o,u)*; "a" is used in front of nouns commencing with a consonant *(letters that are not vowels)* ...DO NOT forget these rules! So, remember we

only use "a"and "an" when we are not talking about one specific thing; that is, about many of the same things. *Next chapter, we talk about using "the".*

3.7 Cross-Cultural Awareness

As was mentioned in Chapter 1, foreigners are very private about their health challenges. When treating a foreign patient, you must always consult him with your prognosis. It is his (patient's) right to determine if he want his family to be aware of the issue.

In western countries, a patient's prognosis is confidential, strictly between the patient and the doctor, no one else, including family.

When treating a foreign patient, you must always consult them with your prognosis; it is their (patient) right to determine if they want their family to be aware of the issue.

3.8 Case Study: Case Presentation and Summary

Sample of Medical Record					
Name and Address of Hospital					
Identification					
		Hospital/Admission Number			
Surname First name Middle name		Gender		Age		Nationality	
Date of birth (DOB)		Marital Status		Occupation		History was given by	
Date of admission			Date of registration		
Full address			Telephone		
Next of kin (NOK)			Address		Contact
Medical History					
Chief complaint (s)					
History of present illness (HPI)					
Review of system (ROS)					
Past medical history / surgical history (PMSHx)					

continued

Medication/Allergy Hx	
Social history (SHx)	
Obstetrics/Gynecology history (OB/Gyn Hx)	
Family history (FHx)	

General Physical Examination

General appearance	
Vital sign (V/S)	T , P, RR, BP
SHEENT (skin, head, ears, eyes, nose and throat)	
Neck	
Back and spine	
Lymph nodes	
Breasts	
Chest: a. Lungs b. Heart	
Abdomen	
Pelvic and genitalia	
Extremities	
Rectal	

Neurological Examination

Mental status: Level of consciousness	Alert, lethargy, semiconscious, coma, deep coma		
Glasgow coma scale (GCS)	**Eye Response** 4 = Open spontaneously 3 = Open to verbal command 2 = Open to pain 1 = No response	**Verbal Response** 5 = Oriented, converses 4 = Disoriented, converses 3 = Inappropriate response 2 = Incomprehensible sounds 1 = No response	**Motor Response** 6 = Obeys commands 5 = Localizes to pain 4 = Withdraws from pain 3 = Decorticate (flex) to pain 2 = Decerebrate (extend) to pain 1 = No response

continued

Orientation	Person, place, time, purpose
Calculation	Memory: a. Recent memory: b. Remote memory:
Language	Spontaneous speech, comprehension, naming, repetition, reading, writing Aphasia (motor aphasia, sensory aphasia, anomic aphasia, mixed aphasia)
Meningeal irritation signs	Neck stiffness, Kernig's sign, Brudzinski's sign
Cranial nerves (CN)	
CN Ⅰ Olfaction	
CN Ⅱ Vision Visual Field Ophthalmoscopic Exam	
CN Ⅲ, Ⅳ, Ⅵ Extraocular movement pupillary response	
CN Ⅴ Facial sensation and muscle of mastication	
CN Ⅶ Facial expression and taste	
CN Ⅷ Hearing and vestibular sense	
• Rinne test • Weber test	
CN Ⅸ Palate evaluation	

continued

CN X Gag reflex and muscle of articulation	
CN XI Sternocleidomastoid and trapezius muscle	
CN XII Tongue Muscle	
Sensory examination: (primary sensation and cortical sensation) Pain (sharp *vs.* dull), temperature (cool *vs.* warm) Vibration and proprioception Light touch and two-point discrimination	

Motor examination:
Muscle bulk
Muscle tone
Muscle strength
	Power: 0–Complete paralysis
	      1–A flicker of contraction only
	      2–Cannot resist gravity, but moves on the bed
	      3–Resists gravity, but cannot resist examiner
	      4–Resists gravity and examiner, but not normal
	      5–Normal power

Reflexes: **Deep tender reflexes** **Superficial reflexes** **Pathological reflexes**	Biceps, triceps, brachioradialis, patellar, and achilles tendon Right: Left: Abdominal cutaneous, cremasteric, bulbocavernous, corneal reflex, anal wink Right: Left: Hoffman, Babinski, Patellar clonus, Ankle clonus, Chaddock, Oppenheim Right: Left:
Others	
Investigations: • X-ray • CT-Scan • MRI • EEG • Angiography	Date of investigation Result

continued

Procedures Lumbar puncture	Date Analysis: WBC Pressure Chloride Magnesium	RBC Calcium Potassium	Glucose Phosphorous	Protein
Assessment	Provisional diagnosis Differential diagnosis Final diagnosis			
Plan				

Summary:

A summary is **usually provided** in **two sentences**.

The first one is one sentence that **summarizes** the important parts of the history-including identifying information, cheif complaint, a **very brief** description of the HPI, plus essential details from the ROS, PMSHx, and FS Hx. The second sentence is a summary of the physical exam findings. You do not need to repeat the specifics of the exam findings if you can briefly summarize them.

Writing Medical Records

4.1 Information Box

Good medical records are one of the cornerstones of efficient and safe clinical care. With the increasing throughput of junior doctors and the evolution of a shift-based hospital staffing system, established techniques for patient handover and properly written medical records are mandatory. Neurosurgical handover and properly written medical records are unique as clinical stories evolve rapidly and patients can not often communicate for themselves. By the time the patient is referred to the neurosurgeon, the story has often been retold many times, and the patient's neurology may have changed. Having a structured approach to telling the patient's story is key. The developing neurosurgeon should quickly decide from the history what the likely diagnosis is, what tests to organize, and what treatment the patient may need. In certain situations, senior doctors may allow students/junior doctors to describe the usual complete history and examination findings considering the generally accepted format. However, if you can identify and summarize these findings, the senior doctor may skip this altogether and ask about investigation and management, thereby allowing more advanced discussion.

This chapter focuses on familiarizing the health professional with vocabulary and terminologies necessary to develop the skill for good medical record writing and providing the opportunities for familiarizing yourself with form and language, which will help facilitate your language and communication skills for good clinical presentation.

4.2 Grammar Tip: the Article "the"

In the last chapter, we discussed the **indefinite articles** *"a"* and *"an"*; in this chapter, we will talk about the **definite article** *"the"*. *"The"* is referred to as the **definite article** because we use it in front of specific nouns in a group; and with something that the reader/listener already knows. Chapter 3, we used this example: *I will see **a** new patient; she was brought in an ambulance a few minutes ago.* The doctor involved would now say: ***The** patient brought in by an ambulance that I just examined has a fractured collar bone.*

We use *"the"* here because we now know what patient the doctor is talking about. Likewise, we would hear a conversation like this:

*Professor, do you remember **the** patient I examined with the fractured collar bone that came into casualty in an ambulance three weeks ago? Well...*

Again ***"the"*** is used here because we are talking about a definite (specific) patient that the doctor discussed before.

There are many times when we can use both an **indefinite article** and the **definite articl** in one sentence:

*I examined **a** patient three weeks ago with a fractured collar bone; well, **the** patient has returned, this time with a broken wrist.*

So do not forget, use an **indefinite article** (a/an) the first time you refer to a noun and use the **definite article** (the) when you refer to the same noun again.

4.3 Cross-Cultural Awareness

It has been said before that western foreigners are direct; this directness applies to writing and speaking. With native English-speaking foreigners, the most important news or information is given first, followed by supporting information; this is called "active language or voice". Overseas, people become impatient with passive language wherein the key information is delivered after all the supporting information is given first. Our advice is to use active voice when giving a foreigner your prognosis; in other words, get straight to the point by saying what is wrong first, then provide all the ancillary information.

4.4 Case Study: Case Presentation

4.4.1 Clinical Presentation

Conveying a clinical presentation can take years of practice. It is an amalgamation of the patient's history, clinical examination, management and current clinical status. It should be delivered concisely and confidently. There is no one "correct way" to do this, and it will vary between clinical specialties, but the following structure is recommended for neurosurgical cases:

1. Introduce the patient

Age, sex, hand dominance, profession, independent and significant comorbidities / relevant drug history. To save time (and words on the handover sheet), you can abbreviate, and in one short line, set the scene and allow your audience to visualize the patient such as the following.

Example: 77-year-old male, right-handed (RH), retired postman, independent, with past medical history (PMHx) of hypertension (HTN) and chronic kidney disease (CKD), on aspirin…

2. Describe the problem

The description of the problem at handover should paint a picture of where the lesion is, what the lesion is and how unwell the patient is. You need to have taken the history and examined the patient yourself to do this correctly.

Example: 51-year-old male, right-handed, builder, co-habits with his wife and children. Witnessed collapse on pavement, no obvious head injury. GCS 8 when the ambulance arrived (M5, V2, E1). En route to hospital fixed and dilated right pupil. GCS 6 on arrival (M4, V1, E1). Intubated and ventilated + mannitol in accident + emergency department, right pupil, remained fixed.

3. Differential Diagnosis

4. Investigations

5. Management

4.4.2 Case Summary and Synthesis

The neurological case is often lengthy and detailed in terms of the complete history and examination findings. It is helpful to routinely summarize the relevant positive and negative findings when writing in the case notes.

This step helps to clarify the case and synthesize the various elements. It should come after the examination findings and consist of just a paragraph or two of the findings. A case summary can be presented during a ward round, turn over round and teaching round. A detailed case presentation can be done when making a case report for discussion in a morning meeting or case discussion seminar.

4.4.3 Neurosurgical Cases

4.4.3.1 Chronic Subdural Hematoma Abbreviations

AF: atrial fibrillation

CSDH: chronic subdural hematoma

CTH: computed tomography head

DVLA: driving and vehicle licensing agency

HTN: hypertension

INR: international normalized ratio (measurement of extrinsic pathway clotting)

RTA: road traffic accident

SAH: sub arachnoid hemorrhage

SDH: subdural hematoma

Clinical Presentation

83-year-old male, right-handed, retired taxi driver, past medical history of HTN and on warfarin for AF, presents with 1 week history of worsening headache and left-side weakness, had a fall at home while entering his bedroom three weeks ago and sustained a mild head injury, on examination GCS 13 (E3, V4, M6), left-sided weakness 4/5, INR 2.6.

Differential Diagnosis

1. CSDH

2. ICH secondary to coagulopathy

3. Aneurysmal SAH with ICH

4. HTN related ICH

The time course of the symptoms is central to distinguishing them: intracerebral hemorrhage (ICH) or stroke typically presents with sudden-onset symptoms; progressive symptoms suggest a slowly enlarging mass such as a tumor or chronic subdural hematoma (CSDH).

Investigations: CTH, CTA

CTH revealed large right convexity sub-acute SDH.

Management

Warfarin reversed with coagulation factors (octaplex) and vitamin K as per hematology, INR 1.2. Two burr hole drainage of right CSDH and subdural drain.

General management: Conservative.

Twist drill craniostomy, single burr hole, two burr holes, mini craniotomy (when significant membrane formation) ± subgaleal or subdural drain.

4.4.3.2 Arteriovenous Malformation Abbreviations

ASDH: acute subdural hematoma

AVM: arteriovenous malformation

CTA: cerebral tomography angiogram

DSA: digital subtraction angiogram

ETOH: alcohol (ethanol alcohol)

EVD: external ventricular drain

h/a: headache

HCP: hydrocephalus

HDU: high dependency unit (area in a hospital, usually close to the intensive care unit for more extensive care but not to the point of intensive care)

HTN: hypertension

ICH: intra-cerebral hematoma

ICP: intra-cranial pressure

MRC grading: Medical Research Council muscle grading

OT: occupational therapy

PT: physiotherapy

SRS: stereotactic radiosurgery

VST: venous sinus thrombosis

Clinical Presentation

17-year-old male, right-handed, student, previously fit and well, while at school suffered sudden severe h/a and subsequent decreased level of consciousness (E1, V1, M5) and right-sided weakness 4/5 MRC grading.

Differential Diagnosis

1. ICH (AVM, HTN, tumor, aneurysm, drugs, EtoH, VST, moyamoya, coagulopathy)

2. Spontaneous ASDH

Investigations: CTH, CTA, DSA

CTH, CTA, DSA revealed left frontal intracerebral hemorrhage with intraventricular extension and hydrocephalus secondary to a ruptured peripheral left frontal AVM.

Management

1. Insertion of right frontal EVD to relieve HCP and control raised ICP.

2. Left pterional craniotomy and excision of AVM.

   – ABCDE protocol assessment (A: airway; B: breathing; C: circulation; D: disability; E: exposure).

   – EVD for HCP or partial evacuation of ICH if patient significantly compromised by raised ICP.

   – Neuro vascular multi-disciplinary team (MDT) as management of AVMs is a multi-modality approach surgery, endovascular therapy, SRS or combination.

4.4.3.3 Spinal Dural Arteriovenous Fistula (SDAVF) Abbreviations

A-V: aterio-venous

L_1: first lumbar vertebrae

MRA: magnetic resonance angiogram

MRI: magnetic resonance imaging

MRI TRICKS: magnetic resonance imaging with time-resolved imaging of contrast kinetics, an MRI sequence that provides MR angiography with an excellent spatial and temporal resolution

MSCC: metastatic spinal cord compression

T_6: sixth thoracic vertebrae

Clinical Presentation

73-year-old female, a retired pharmacist, past medical history of lymphedema and bilateral hip replacements, presents with four months history of gradually worsening mobility and sphincteric dysfunction. One month to presentation had more rapid deterioration and double incontinence and unsteadiness one week to presentation. She had lower thoracic severe myelopathy on examination with loss of proprioception, weakness 4/5, double incontinence, and can feel catheter tug.

Differential Diagnosis

1. Thoracic spine MSCC

2. Thoracic spine meningioma

3. Thoracic disc prolapse or stenosis

4. Thoracic dural A-V fistula

5. Inflammatory/demyelination process

Investigations: MRI, MRI TRICKS

MRI spine revealed cord signal change consistent with edema secondary to venous hypertension from T_6 to L_1 and numerous punctate flow voids predominantly at T_9-T_{10}, appearances consistent with dural arteriovenous fistula.

MRI supplemented with TRICKS sequence/DSA, which demonstrated early filling caudally directed draining vein with the point of fistulation likely at T_8 level on the left, which was confirmed with selective spinal catheter angiogram.

Management

Underwent uneventful T_8 laminectomy and disconnection of dural A-V fistula. Post-operative imaging with MRI/MRA/DSA confirmed no residual A-V shunting and improvement of cord edema.

4.4.3.4　Craniopharyngioma Abbreviations

MDT: multi-disciplinary team

T_1WI: T_1 weighted MRI imaging sequence

T_1WI + C(Gd): T_1 weighted MRI imaging sequence with contrast (gadolinium)

T_2WI: T_2 weighted MRI imaging sequence

Clinical Presentation

58-year-old male with short stature presented with 3 months history of blurred vision. The ophthalmologist routine eye screen highlighted reduced visual acuity (6/60), associated with photophobia, and a mild headache, no history of vomiting, seizures, polyuria or polydipsia; no family history of brain tumors. On examination, GCS 15/15, bitemporal hemianopia.

Differential Diagnosis Sellar/suprasellar lesion

1. Craniopharyngioma
2. Meningioma
3. Hypothalamic harmatoma
4. Pituitary macroadenoma (with cystic degeneration or necrosis)

Investigations: MRI

1. T_1WI: cysts iso to hyperintense to the brain (due to high protein content "machinery oil cysts").
2. T_2WI: variable, but ~80% are mostly or partly T_2WI hyperintense.
3. Solid component: T_1WI +C (Gd), vivid enhancement; T_2WI, variable or mixed.

Management

1. Pituitary hormone profile
2. Endocrine advice
3. Insertion of lumbar drain and transsphenoidal resection of sellar/suprasellar lesion (image-guided)

Histology: adamantinomatous craniopharyngioma, with no evidence of atypia

4.4.3.5　Glioma Abbreviations

C/o: complaining of

D: Days

GTR: gross total resection

HGG: high-grade glioma

PPI: proton pump inhibitor

UMN: upper motor neuron

Clinical Presentation

60-year-old female, previously healthy and still very active, non-smoker, lives with her husband, presented with a four-week history of right-sided facial and limb weakness and focal seizure activity after two days of behavioral change and mild cognitive decline. Currently no complaint of a headache, intact neurologically except mild cognitive impairment and subtle right UMN facial weakness, no speech impairment or pronator drifts.

Differential Diagnosis

1. Left frontal/temporal tumor (glioma, metastasis, meningioma)
2. Left sided CSDH
3. Intracranial infection (abscess)
4. Left sided cerebral infarction

Investigations: MRI

MRI brain revealed left insular HGG.

Management

Commence on anti-epileptic and steroid therapy with PPI cover; undergo neuro-psychology assessment and preoperative navigated transcranial magnetic stimulation for motor and speech mapping followed by sharp image-guided craniotomy with neuromonitoring.

4.4.3.6 Meningioma Abbreviations

ACA: anterior cerebral artery

AqS: aqueductal stenosis

Hx: history

NPH: normal pressure hydrocephalus

PMHx: past medical history

SOL: space occupying lesion

Clinical Presentation

61-year-old male, lives with wife, ex-smoker (stopped five years ago), no other significant PMHx, presents with 1-year Hx of gradually worsening h/a, behavioral changes and vacant episodes (absent seizures) on a background of 3-year anosmia. On examination, he had mild cognitive impairment and short-term memory deficit and anosmia.

Differential Diagnosis

1. Frontal neoplastic SOL (extra-axial: meningioma, intra axial: glioma)

2. NPH, longstanding HCP from AqS

3. Dementia

Investigations: MRI

MRI brain revealed olfactory groove meningioma with associated peri-tumoral edema.

Management

Administration of steroids with PPI cover and anti-epileptics. A preoperative CTA is often performed to document the relationship of the ACAs to the tumor.

Undergo elective bifrontal craniotomy and resection of olfactory groove meningioma.

4.4.3.7 Brain Metastasis Abbreviations

CT CAP: computed tomography chest abdomen and pelvis

M: months

MDT: multi-disciplinary team

Mets: metastasis

PF: posterior fossa

RF EVD: right frontal external ventricular drain

TNM: tumor node metastasis cancer grading system

SCC: squamous cell carcinoma

Clinical Presentation

61-year-old male lives with a friend, ex-smoker, has a background history of hypopharynx SCC (T_{4A}, N_{2C}, M_0), resected one year ago followed by adjuvant chemoradiotherapy, presents with a one-month history of h/a, ataxia, left-sided dysmetria and visual impairment secondary to papilledema and deteriorates rapidly to GCS Eye Opening 2 Vocal Tracheostomy Motor 4. No fever and no neck stiffness.

Differential Diagnosis

1. HCP secondary to PF metastatic disease or carcinomatous meningitis

2. Multiple intracranial metastases

3. Intracranial infection due to immunosuppression

4. Intracranial hemorrhage due to treatment-related coagulopathy

Investigations: CTH, MRI, CT CAP

Urgent CTH pre and post-contrast revealed HCP secondary to left cerebellum metastasis,

MRI confirmed solitary deposit, CT CAP excluded metastatic disease elsewhere.

Management

Perform urgent insertion of RF EVD to relieve the HCP and recover the GCS. Commence on high-dose steroids with PPI cover, which can be gradually weaned down post-operatively. Since there is no disease elsewhere, MDT should resect cerebellar metastasis through PF craniectomy. Subsequently, EVD should be removed 72 hours after.

4.4.3.8 Pituitary Adenoma Abbreviations

ACTH: adrenocorticotropic hormone

FSH: follicle-stimulating hormone

GH: growth hormone

HCP: hydrocephalus

IGF-I: insulin-like growth factor

Na: sodium

N/V: nausea and vomiting

PRL: prolactin

SAH: subarachnoid hemorrhage

T_4: thyroxine

TDS: three times daily

TSH: thyroid-stimulating hormone

VF: visual fields

Clinical Presentation

56-year-old male, right-handed, non-smoker, lives with wife and two children, no significant PMHx, reports libido loss over the last 6 months, presents with sudden severe h/a associated with neck pain, n/v, and blurred vision. On examination, he was drowsy but oriented and obeying commands with bitemporal hemianopia and visual acuity right 6/12 (corrected, glasses).

Differential Diagnosis

1. Pituitary apoplexy (adenoma)

2. Craniopharyngioma with HCP

3. Aneurysmal SAH

Investigations: The Pituitary Profile, Formal VF, CTH, CTA, Brain MRI

CTH revealed pituitary apoplexy secondary to suprasellar lesion, most likely adenoma. Note expansion and thinning of bony sella consistent with pituitary adenoma.

CTA ruled out underlying vascular abnormality.

MRI confirmed pituitary macroadenoma with hemorrhagic and necrotic components secondary to apoplexy and compression of the optic chiasm.

Management

- After pituitary profile sent from peripheral blood, commence on steroid replacement therapy with hydrocortisone 100mg TDS.
- Endoscopic transnasal transphenoidal resection of pituitary adenoma.

General

- Pituitary adenomas usually present with VF deficit and hormone oversecretion (PRL: amenorrhea-galactorrhea-loss of libido; GH: acromegaly; ACTH: Cushing's; TSH: hyperthyroidism) or panhypopituitarism.
- Also, it can cause h/a from dural irritation secondary to diaphragm sella stretching.
- Pituitary profile includes: 8 a.m. cortisol, 24 hours urine free cortisol, T_4, TSH, PRL, FSH, LH, IGF-I, fasting blood glucose.
- Prolactinoma can be managed with dopamine agonists (bromocriptine, cabergoline), acromegaly with dopamine agonists, somatostatin analog (octreotide), GH antagonist (pegvisomant), Cushing's with ketoconazole, metyrapone.

4.4.3.9 Cerebral Abscess Abbreviations

Abx: antibiotics

i.v.: intra venous

MRI DWI: diffusion-weighted magnetic resonance imaging (looks at the restricted movement of hydrogen molecules and is useful in identifying infarct, intracerebral abscess and tumors with high cellularity)

Clinical Presentation

25-year-old male, student, non-smoker, previously healthy, presents with a one-week history of right periorbital cellulitis, was commenced on oral abx at the community, admitted urgently into the local hospital with pyrexia, confusion and drowsiness, deteriorated rapidly to GCS 8 (E2, V2, M4) with left side hemisphere, fixed and dilated right pupil. Intravenous access was established urgently, and hyperosmotic therapy with mannitol commenced and blue lighted (like Chinese green-lighted) to the neurosurgical operating theatre.

Differential Diagnosis

1. Intracranial infection (extradural abscess, subdural empyema, intracerebral abscess).

2. Pott's puffy tumor.

Investigations: CTH

CTH revealed right-sided subdural empyema and extradural abscess causing mass effect secondary to frontal sinusitis and periorbital cellulitis (note that imaging usually underestimates extent of subdural empyema).

Management

Undergo urgent right-sided fronto-temporal craniectomy for evacuation of extradural abscess and subdural empyema plus Fiber optic endoscopic sinus surgery by transnasal approach. Surgery and washout of Frontal Sinus followed by 6 weeks administration of i.v. abx therapy ceftriaxone and vancomycin (most common pathogen is streptococcus milleri) also commence on prophylactic anti-epileptic (phenytoin) therapy since intracranial infection imposes high risk of epilepsy 40%-80%.

Special Medical Documentations

5.1 Information Box

For more than a century, health records were created and maintained in paper-based formats. However, most nations have been experiencing a transformation from paper-based health care documents to digital documents in recent years. To develop an electronic medical record, an electronic representation of the paper documents must be determined. Several different terms have been used to describe computer-based records. Today, **electronic health record (EHR)** is the term used most widely. Other terms used most commonly include **electronic medical record (EMR)** and **computer-based patient record (CPR)**. When a hospital is transitioning from paper to an electronic system and uses both components, the record is a **hybrid health record**. A health record is a tool used by patient's caregivers to communicate with each other. The records maintained by health care providers for patients, no matter the illness or health care setting, contain similar information. However, some settings and medical specialties have specific documentation requirements that are unique to their field. This chapter provides young English second language health professionals opportunities to familiarize themselves with the common types of paper-based format of frequently used medical documents in neurosurgery.

5.2 Grammar Tip: Singular and Plural

When speaking, particularly writing English, a common misunderstanding is called *'singular* and *plural'* referring to nouns and verbs. The determination of whether a noun is *singular* or *plural* depends upon that nouns countability; if the noun can be counted, as in-hospital patients, then both the singular and pleural can apply: *I will see a patient at 7:30, while my professors will see seven patients in the morning.* Because we can count the number of *'patients',* it can be *singular* (one only) or *plural* (two or more).

For non-native English speakers, confusion arises over two key issues: knowing what nouns are countable and which are not. *'Water'*, for example, is uncountable in any language. *'Furniture'* in many languages is countable, but not in English, so it is uncountable so stays singular. *'Furniture'* in English is called a general or broad term that includes many parts like 'chairs' 'beds' 'tables'; these parts are of course countable, and can be plural; but, *'furniture'* itself is uncountable. some nouns have no logic as to why they are only singular; you have to learn these.

How to show a noun is plural

In most cases, we add /-s/ to the end of the countable noun to indicate plurality; however, you need to know the exceptions to this rule.

Noun ending in:	Make plural by:	Examples
ch, sh, ss, x, zz	adding–es	lunch–lunches
y	dropping the y and adding–ies	baby–babies
f or fe	dropping the f or fe and adding–ves	knife–knives

Next Chapter, we discuss plural and singular verbs.

5.3　Culture Awareness

This cultural awareness element is one that nothing, if little, can be done about, but one that you need to be aware of. In China, in a clinic, doctors have many patients to see; as a result, they can only allocate perhaps less than 30 minutes for each person. Foreigners may find this worrying as they are probably used to longer consultation periods in their homeland.

The speed of the visit coupled with the continual interruptions by other patients can cause the foreign patient to become irritable. In such a situation many first-time foreign visitors feel like being in a factory machine and can not relax throughout the visit. Should you notice that your foreign patient appears anxious about the environment, assure them that you will provide them with the best possible attention.

5.4　Consultation Request Note

It is a common practice that the diagnosis or treatment of certain cases requires the joint effort of a multi-disciplinary team. Accurate communication between the **referring physician** and the **consulting physician** is needed for effective consultation and collaboration between physicians. A consultation request note should contain the patient's information, clinical condition, the existing problem and relevant investigations results; the reason or purpose of consultation should also be clarified.

Name and Address of Hospital Medical Consultation Request

Patient's data:		
Name: Age: Sex: Hosp.#: Bed#:		
From: _____ Please return to the above address		
To:_____		

Purpose/reasons for consultation:

Provisional diagnosis:

Clinical information:

Signature: _____   Date: _____

Referring physician

Physician's response:

Signature: _____   Date: _____

Consulting physician

5.5 Informed Consent

Informed consent is a communication process between the health care provider and the patient that often leads to agreement or permission for care, treatment, or service. Every patient has the right to get information and ask questions before procedures and treatment. If adult patients can make their own decisions, medical care cannot begin unless they give informed consent.

Name and Address of Hospital Informed Consent

Patient's data:
Name: Age: Sex: Hosp.#:
Address: Phone #:
This consent provides us with permission to perform reasonable and necessary medical examinations and treatment. By signing below, you are indicating that: 1. You intend this consent to continue in nature even after a specific diagnosis has been made and treatment recommended 2. You consent to treatment at this hospital. This consent will remain fully effective until it is revoked in writing *I voluntarily request a physician and mid-level provider (nurse, practitioner, physician assistant, or clinical nurse specialist), and other health care providers or the designees as necessary, to perform reasonable and necessary medical examinations, testing and treatment for the condition which has brought me to seek care at this practice.*
I _____ certify that I have fully understood the above statement and consent fully and voluntarily to its contents.

_____   _____
    Signature of patient   Date
 	
_____   _____
    Name of relative   Relationship to patient
 	
_____   _____
    Signature of witness   Date

5.6 Operative Notes/Operative Report

Operative Report or Note is the document to record the surgical procedure by the surgeon. In brief, a quality Operative Note should contain sufficient information to identify the patient, support or modify the pre-operative diagnosis, and to justify the surgical procedure performed. In Neurosurgery, there is other documentation necessary to be completed.

In addition to the pre-operative note and the post-operative note, the patient needs to sign a neurosurgery consent form; the risk assessment form and safety check form need to be completed as well; the blood request form needs to be filled out to prepare blood for intra-operative or post-operative transfusion; finally, a pathology request form needs to be completed for intra-operative or post-operative pathologic evaluation.

Physician: _____
Procedure: _____
Date: _____
□ Confirmed identity of the patient
□ The confirmed medical record is for the correct patient
□ Authentic images are for the correct patient
□ Confirmed the correct operation
□ Confirmed that consent form is signed for the correct operation
□ Antibiotic was given as ordered
Signature of surgeon completing the checklist: _____

5.6.1 Pre-Operative and Post-Operative Note

Morbidity due to avoidable medical errors is a crippling reality intrinsic to health care. In particular, iatrogenic surgical errors lead to significant morbidity, decreased quality of life, and attendant costs. In recent decades there has been an increased focus on health care quality improvement, with an accompanying focus on mitigating avoidable medical errors. The unique tool developed to this end is the surgical checklist. Checklists have been implemented in various operating rooms internationally, with overwhelmingly positive results.

General neurological pre-operative checklist Post-operative note

Name and Address of Hospital Operative Report

Patient's name: Age: Sex: Hosp.#:   Bed#:

Date: _____ Time Start: _____ End: _____

Pre-operative diagnosis: _____

Post-operative diagnosis: _____

Procedure: _____

Surgeon: _____

Assistants:1. _____ 2. _____ 3. _____

Anesthesia: _____

Anesthesiologist: _____

Description of procedure:

Findings:

Specimen:

Inputs/Outputs:

Estimated blood loss (EBL):

Unrine output (UOP):

Intra venous fluids:

Drain (s):

Complications:

Condition:

Name: _____ Signature: _____ Date: _____

(Name, Title)

5.6.2 Neurosurgery Informed Consent Form

Name and Address of Hospital Neurosurgery Informed Consent Form

Patient's name: Age: Sex: Hosp.#:   Bed#:

Clinical Diagnosis: _____

Procedure (s): _____

Date: _____ Address: _____

continued

According to the patient's condition, existing symptoms and relevant examinations, the patient was diagnosed with _____. For appropriate management, the attending physician has suggested surgical treatment on ____ Month ____ Day ____ Year ____. Surgery is a high-risk and difficult treatment. Given the limitations of current medical science and technology, individual specificity of patients, differences in disease conditions, age and other factors, safe surgery without any risk doesn't exist. Due to known and unforeseen reasons, the operation may be a failure, have complications, injury of adjacent organs or some incidents that are difficult to prevent and deal with. Even if the medical staff have conscientiously done their duty and diligently carried out their services, the following medical risks may still occur during the operation:

1. Anesthesia accident, cardiac arrest, respiratory arrest and other life-threatening conditions.

2. The surgery might result in failure of important functional areas or important cerebral vessels or nerves, uncontrollable bleeding and acute brain swelling may occur during the operation, which may lead to failure of the operation, or cause shock, respiratory and circulatory failure and endanger life.

3. Intracranial hematoma, cerebral edema, hydrocephalus, cerebral infarction or intraspinal hemorrhage may occur after the surgery. If the medical treatment is unsuccessful, the patient will need to be operated on again. If the rescue fails, it may endanger life.

4. Postoperative neurological dysfunction may occur, including disturbance of consciousness, hemiplegia, aphasia, sensory impairment, loss of smell, hemianopia, vision loss, blindness, eyelid and eye movement disorders (such as strabismus, diplopia, etc.), facial numbness or pain, corneal ulcer, facial paralysis, hearing loss or deafness, hoarseness, dysphagia, dyspnea (even with the need for tracheotomy) may occur. Severe disturbance of respiratory and circulatory function may endanger life; serious damage to the hypothalamus may lead to diabetes insipidus, gastrointestinal bleeding, electrolyte and metabolic disorder, intractable hyperglycemia, high fever, coma, etc.; mental disorder, dementia, epilepsy, ataxia, long-term coma, survival only to a vegetative state, etc. may occur in the later stage.

5. Spinal cord surgery can lead to paraplegia, quadriplegia, limb numbness, hypoesthesia or loss of body deep sensation, defecation and sexual dysfunction, dyspnea or severe dyspnea, and even death. The spine's stability can be affected, resulting in late spinal distortion, which might need to be corrected again.

6. Shunt blockage, implant rejection, or infection in ventriculoperitoneal shunt (VPS), external ventricular drainage (EVD), and cranioplasty. Reoperation might be required, and the shunt or artificial skull might need to be removed. The spread of inflammation and recurrence of an abscess may occur after the operation of a brain abscess. Transsphenoidal surgery may cause cerebrospinal fluid rhinorrhea, nasal septum defect, nasal mucosa atrophy, rhinitis, epistaxis and other complications.

7. Most tumors of the brain and spinal cord are malignant growth, which may not be completely removed after surgery, and other treatments should be supplemented post-surgery; even benign lesions (such as meningioma, pituitary tumor, neurilemmoma, vascular malformation, etc.) that are located deep or adjacent to important structures, they may not be completely removed. The initial symptoms may not be improved or might even worsen and recur in the future.

continued

a. Aneurysm rupture may occur during aneurysm surgery, causing massive bleeding, shock, coagulation mechanism disorder, leading to life-threatening risk; aneurysm clipping is not a complete solution. There can be a recurrence, rebleeding, aneurysm clip-off, which might need to be re-clipped; if the aneurysm can not be clipped during the operation, other surgical methods should be adopted.

b. After surgery, disturbance of consciousness, limb paralysis, aphasia, epilepsy and mental retardation may occur due to cranial nerve injury or cerebral vasospasm; there may also be vision loss or blindness, visual field damage, eyelid ptosis, strabismus, diplopia, hoarseness, dysphagia. The main purpose of aneurysm surgery is to prevent rebleeding and saveth life of the patient. However, serious consequences and secondary reactions such as vasospasm and hydrocephalus might still need further treatment.

8. The operation may be complicated with intracranial infection, incision site infection, poor wound healing, cerebrospinal fluid leakage, respiratory tract and urinary tract infection, and septicemia. Intracranial infection and cerebrospinal fluid leakage, repeated lumbar puncture or lumbar puncture and drainage, or even secondary surgery will increase hospitalization time and expenses.

The above situations are likely to occur, the patient and/or family could incur aggravation or even life-threatening, and its corresponding economic burden: the physician has given me and/or us a detailed description of the situation, and I and/or we acknowledge the circumstances associated with the surgery and the risks or complications that may occur during the surgery.

Patient or relative: _____ (Relationship to patient): _____

Doctor: _____ Attending (or senior) doctor: _____ Date: _____

5.6.3 Surgical Risks Assessment Form

Name of Hospital Surgical Risks Assessment Form

Department: _____ Patient's name: _____ Age:_____

Sex:_____ Hosp.#: _____ Bed#: _____

Procedure: _____

continued

Anesthesia grading (ASA classification)	**P1**	There was no systemic disease except local lesions	0
	P2	The patient had mild clinical symptoms and mild or moderate systemic diseases	0
	P3	Severe systemic disease, limited daily activities, but no loss of work ability	1
	P4	Have serious systemic disease, have lost the ability to work, threaten life safety	1
	P5	Critically ill, life-threatening patients	1
	P6	Patients with brain death	1
Signature of anesthesiologist		_____ Month _____ Day _____ Year	
Surgical incision cleanliness	**Type Ⅰ surgical incision** (clean surgery)	■ There was no pollution in the surgical field and no inflammation around the incision ■ The patient not intubated, no esophagus and urethra catheter inserted ■ The patient has no disturbance of consciousness	0
	Type Ⅱ surgical incision (relatively clean operation)	■ Procedures involving the upper and lower respiratory tract, upper and lower digestive tract, urogenital tract or any surgery through the above organs ■ Intubation, esophagus and urethra catheter inserted ■ The patient's condition is stable ■ Patients undergoing gallbladder, vagina, appendix, ear and nose surgery	0
	Type Ⅲ surgical incision (clean contamination surgery)	■ Open, fresh and unclean wounds ■ Incision with infection after the previous operation ■ Incision requiring disinfection during operation	1

continued

	Type Ⅳ surgical incision (contaminated surgery)	■ Severe trauma with inflammation, tissue necrosis, or visceral drainage tube	1
Estimated operative duration	T1: the operation is expected to be completed within 3 hours		0
	T2: the operation is expected to be completed in more than 3 hours		1
Category of surgery	Superficial tissue surgery		
	Deep tissue surgery		
	Organ surgery		
	Lacunar surgery		
Preoperative NNIS classification	Anesthesia ASA grading + surgical incision cleanliness + duration of surgery = 0 - 1 - 2 - 3-		
Signature of surgeon	_____ Month _____ Day _____ Year		
Emergency (yes/no)	**Emergency surgery**		
Estimated operative duration	T1: the operation is expected to be completed within 3 hours		0
	T2: the operation is expected to be completed in more than 3 hours		1
Postoperative NNIS grading	Anesthesia ASA grading + surgical incision cleanliness + duration of surgery = 0 - 1 - 2 - 3-		
Signature of circulating nurse	_____ Month _____ Day _____ Year		
Wound healing	Primary healing Superficial wound infection Deep wound infection Others _____		
Signature of attending physician	_____ Month _____ Day _____ Year		

5.6.4 Surgical Safety Check List

Name of Hospital Surgical Safety Checklist

Department: _____ Patient's name: _____ Age: _____

Sex: _____ Bed#: _____ Hosp.#: _____

Anesthesia: _____ Surgeon:_____ Procedure: _____ Date: _____

Before induction of anaesthesia: SIGN IN	**Before skin incision: TIME OUT**	**Before the patient leaves the operating room: SIGN OUT**
PATIENT HAS CONFIRMED • Identity • Site • Procedure • Consent	Confirmed all team members have introduced themselves by name and role	**THE NURSE VERBALLY CONFIRMED WITH THE TEAM:** The name of the procedure recorded That instrument, sponge and needle counts are correct (or not applicable) How the specimen is labeled (including patient name)

SITE MARKED/NOT APPLICABLE	Surgeon, anaesthesia professional and nurse verbally confirm:
	    Patient
	    Site
	    Procedure	

ANAESTHESIA SAFETY CHECK COMPLETED	ANTICIPATED CRITICAL EVENTS: **SURGEON REVIEWS:** What are the unexpected critical steps, operative duration, anticipated blood loss?	Whether there are any equipment problems to be addressed
PULSE OXIMETER ON PATIENT AND FUNCTIONING	**ANAESTHESIA TEAM REVIEW:** Are there any patient-specific concerns? **NURSING TEAM REVIEWS:** Has sterility (including indicator results) been confirmed? Are there equipment issues or any concern?	Surgeon, anaesthesia, professional and nurse review the key concerns for recovery and management of the patient

continued

DOES THE PATIENT HAS A: KNOW ALLERGY? No Yes DIFFICULT AIRWAY/ ASPIRATION RISK No Yes, and Equipment /Assistant available risk of >500ml Blood loss (7ml/kg in children)? No Yes, and adequate intravenous access and fluids planned	**HAS ANTIBIOTIC PROPHYLAXIS BEEN GIVEN WITHIN THE LAST 60 MINUTES?** Yes Not applicable **IS ESSENTIAL IMAGING DISPLAYED?** Yes Not applicable	Surgeon, anaesthesia, professional and nurse review the key concerns for recovery and management of the patient

5.6.5 Blood Transfusion Request Form

Clinical Blood Transfusion Application Form

Scheduled date of blood transfusion: _____ Month _____ Day _____ Year

Name of recipient: _____ Gender: _____ age: _____

Hospital #.: _____ Department: _____ Bed #: _____

Clinical diagnosis: _____

Purpose of blood transfusion: _____

Indications of blood transfusion: _____

Previous blood transfusion history: ① yes; ② no (please tick √ for selection)

Recipient's territory: ① this city; ② areas outside the city (please tick √)

Signing of blood transfusion consent: ① yes; ② no (reason for not signing:)

Scheduled blood transfusion components: _____

Scheduled blood transfusion volume: _____

Nature of blood transfusion: ① emergency; ② routine; ③ standby; ④ intraoperative reserve
(please tick √)

Before blood transfusion, laboratory tests should be performed:

ABO blood group: _____ Rh: _____ Hemoglobin: _____ g / L HCT: _____ %

platelet: _____ $\times 10^9$ / L

continued

ALT: _____ U/L   HBsAg: _____

Anti-HCV: _____ Anti-HIV1/2: _____ Syphilis: _____

Signature of applying physician: _____

Signature of attending physician: _____

Application date: _____ Month _____ Day _____ Year

(Note: please fill in item by item carefully and accurately, and send it to the blood transfusion department/blood bank before the date of blood transfusion)

5.6.6 Pathology Request Form

The pathologist plays an essential role in patient care as a diagnostician, patient advocate, and clinical teacher. The surgical pathologist examines tissues and foreign objects extracted from patients to identify disease processes. Specimens submitted for examinations include fluids, cells and tissues. It is the responsibility of the hospital personnel involved to ensure that each patient's specimen is appropriately and safely handled and processed. When a pathologist examination is requested, the following information must be provided: patients identification (patient's name, sex, age, hospital number) and good clinical history. The format of a standard pathology report includes gross examination/gross description, image, final diagnosis and immunohistochemical stain, date and signature of the pathologist.

Name of Hospital Pathology Examination Request and Reporting Form

Patient's name: _____ Age: _____ Sex: _____ Bed#: _____

Date submitted: _____ Date received: _____ Requesting department: _____

Clinical diagnosis:

Clinical history:

Type of specimen:

continued

Findings during operation:

Gross description and:

Image:

Final diagnosis:

Immunohistochemical stain:

Report date: ____ Month ____ Day ____ Year

Signature of pathologist:

5.7 Prescriptions Form and Doctor's Order

Prescriptions and doctor's medication orders are the primary means the prescribers communicate with the pharmacists regarding the desired treatment regimen for the patient. Prescriptions are used in the outpatient, or ambulatory setting, whereas medication orders are used in the inpatient or institutional health setting. Prescriptions and inpatient orders are legal orders that can be used for medications, devices, laboratory tests, procedures, and the like. Prescriptions and medication orders can be handwritten, typed, pre-printed, verbal or entered into a computer program and submitted to the pharmacy by the patient or caregivers.

Medication orders typically contain similar information that would be included on a prescription. This includes the patient's name and a second identifier such as patient's date of birth and medical record number; the patient's location and room number;

date and time of order; the drug name, dose, route, frequency, and duration; and the prescriber's name and signature.

Name of Hospital Prescription Form

Patient's name: _____ Age: _____ Sex: _____ Bed#: _____   Hospital #: _____ Department: _____ Clinical diagnosis: _____ Date _____   Address/Contact #:
Rx: **Vancomycin 1,500mg, I.V.,q.12hours × 3days**   **Name and signature of the physician:** _____ **License #:** _____   **Name and signature of pharmacist:** _____

Name of Hospital

Doctor's order

Patient's name: _____ Age: _____ Sex: _____ Bed#: _____
Hospital #: _____ Department: _____ Clinical diagnosis: _____ Date _____

Date	Order	Prescriber
08/31/2020 @ 8:15a.m.	**Vancomycin 1,500mg. i.v., q.12hours × 3days**	Dr. A.K. Ballah
08/31/2020 @ 9:15a.m.	Remove Folley catheter	Dr. A.K. Ballah

5.8 Progress Notes

Progress notes are the part of a medical record where the health care professionals record and document a patient's clinical status during hospitalization or throughout outpatient care.

Progress notes are written in various formats depending on the situation and the information the clinician wishes to record. One example is the **SOAP** note, organized into **subjective, objective, assessment and plan** sections. Another example is the **DART** system, organized into **description, assessment, response and treatment**.

Both physicians and nurses write progress notes to document patient care regularly during a patient's hospitalization.

Name of Hospital

Doctor's Progress Note	
Patient's name: _____ Hospital#: _____	
Date & Time	

Signature and Title Must Appear After Each Entry

5.9 Referral Form

A doctor referral form is a form that physicians need to fill in and sign before referring a patient to a specialist for better treatment and diagnosis.

Name and Address of Hospital Referral Form

Patient's data: Name: Age: Sex: Hosp.#:   DOB#: From: _____ Please return to the above address To: _____
Purpose/reasons for referral:
Provisional diagnosis:
Clinical information:

continued

Name and signature: _____ Date: _____	
	Referring physician
Office contact contact person: _____ Office address: _____	
Phone #: _____ Fax#: _____	
Please attach supporting medical documents (last office note, medical history, labs and medications)	

5.10 Discharge Note/Discharge Summary

A hospital discharge summary is a very important medical document. It summarizes the patient's clinical status during hospitalization and written communication to the post-discharge medical setting. It provides professional instructions for patients and their relatives. The documented information should be concise, and important elements should be included. The following items are the most important components that should be contained in a well-written discharge summary: patient's information, diagnosis (both on admission and discharge), the reason for hospitalization, significant findings, treatment provided, discharge condition, and post-discharge instruction.

Name and Address of Hospital Discharge Summary

Patient's name: _____ Age: _____ Sex: _____ Bed#: _____ Hospital#: _____ Discharging department: _____ Date of admission: _____
Date of discharge: Admission diagnosis: Discharge diagnosis:
Reasons for hospitalization:
Laboratory data:
Important consultation:
Pathological findings:

continued

Treatment provided:
Complications:
Discharge condition:
Discharge medication:
Discharge /follow-up instruction:
      Name and signature: _____ Date: _____
         Attending physician

5.11 Medical Report

A medical report is a comprehensive report that covers a person's clinical history. A medical report is an updated detail of a medical examination of a certain patient. It is a vital and written document that describes the findings of an individual or group of people. A medical report should contain accurate and credible data.

Name and Address of Hospital Medical Report

Name: Age: Sex: Hosp.#:   DOB#: RE: _____
Background:
Medical history:
Examination:
Specimens:
Management:

Opinion:
     Name and signature: _____ Date: _____
        Attending physician

5.12 Death Certificate, Morbidity and Mortality Review

World Health Organization has a standardized medical certification of cause of death with instructions for physicians and surgeons to complete with a recommended international standard.

I	(a)	Approximate interval between onset and death
Disease or condition directly leading to death*	Due to (or as a consequence of)	
	(b)	
	Due to (or as a consequence of)	
Antecedent causes Morbid conditions, if any, giving rise to the above cause, stating the underlying condition last	(c)	
	Due to (or as a consequence of)	
	(d)	
	Due to (or as a consequence of)	
II		
Other significant conditions contributing to the death, but not related to the disease or condition causing it		
*This does not mean the mode of dying, e.g. heart failure, respiratory failure. It means the disease, injury, or complication that caused death.		

Writing Case Report

6.1 Information Box

Writing a case report is like writing a detective story. There must be a problem that needs a solution, some kind of intrigue to keep the readers interested in the situation and enough information for the readers to understand the problem. A medical case study report is an article that describes a particular patient's diagnosis and treatment plan. Most of the cases chosen for medical case studies are of unusual diagnoses or include complications in treatment. A case study report is written in a specific format and can be submitted to peer-reviewed journals. To write a medical case study report you will need to partner with a supervising physician and colleagues, collect information about the patient and obtain the proper consent to write and publish the report.

6.2 Grammar Tip: Subject Verb Agreement

Many of you will have studied what is called subject verb agreement in school.

To refresh your memories, the subject verb agreement means that if you use a singular (one only) noun in the subject of a sentence, you must use a singular verb.

Example:

The doctor is/are operating now.

"Doctor" is the singular subject, and "is" is the Singular verb, so we must use "is". We use "are" if the Subject is plural...

The doctors is/are operating now.

This seems simple enough, but often there is a mistake with regular verbs like "work""operate ""run" and so on.

Many students believe that to make a plural noun; we generally add /-s/to the end of the noun; therefore, we do the same with regular verbs.

NOT SO! A plural noun has /-s/, a singular noun has no /-s/; conversely, a plural verb has no /-s/, yet a singular verb does.

The doctor operates every day.

Singular subject = "doctor "+ singular verb= "operates "(notice the /-s/ on the end of the singular verb).

The doctors operate every day.

Plural subject ="doctors" + plural verb= "operate" (notice no /-s/ on the end of the plural verb).

Remember: singular verb **add** /-s/ and plural verb **no** /-s/.

6.3 Cross-Cultural Awareness

A hard truth about many foreigners is a lack of respect for titles; this is particularly true of Australians. This does not mean that they lack respect for educated people; just because someone is called a "professor" means little to them. Respect comes from what they can do, not their title.

I raise this because a recent incident in a local hospital was brought to my attention involving a Chinese professor and a German. A relatively young Chinese doctor treated the German when a Chinese professor wanted to take over. The German became angry at the professor and insisted that the younger doctor keep going with whom he could talk. The professor (via an English-speaking nurse) said she was a "professor" and could do better than the young doctor. The German was becoming angrier and said he did not care what the professor called herself; she could not speak English, so he didn't want her to treat him. Of course, the German was wrong, in the Chinese context; but take note that foreigners base their level of respect on what a person does and if they can communicate, not what they are called.

6.4 Principles of Writing Medical Case Report

There are five steps to write a medical case study report.

Step1: Select a Case

- Be aware of patients who have a rare or unusual illness. These are the types of cases that are often selected for publication. Also, pay attention to treatments that have an expected positive or negative outcome.
- Speak with senior physicians about patients whose illness would make an interesting case study report. Senior physicians can be a valuable source of information. They may have notes for reports for which they need assistance writing. You may also want to choose additional colleagues to contribute to the report.

The selected case must meet one of the following criteria:

1. Unreported or unusual side effects or adverse interactions involving medications.

2. Unexpected or unusual presentations of a disease.

3. New associations or variation in disease processes.

4. Presentations, diagnoses and management of new and emerging disease.

5. An unexpected association between diseases or symptoms.

6. An unexpected event in the course of observing or treating a patient.

7. Findings that shed new light on the possible pathogenesis of a disease or an adverse effect.

Step 2: Research the Case

- Review the current literature on the diagnosis or treatment that will focus on your case study report. Seek assistance from your hospital's library staff. Librarians can help you find journal articles or books that provide the most current information on your topic of interest. This information will be a significant part of your paper once you begin writing.

Step 3: Collect Patient Information and Consent

- Medical ethics requires that the patient who is the focus of your medical case study report provides written consent. Many journals have their consent forms that the patient must complete and sign before you submit your report.

- Gather the patient's demographic information (age, medical history, medication use, current and past diagnoses, etc.). Provide detailed information about the patients so your audience will be well informed about the case.

- Collect copies of the patient's labs, X-rays or any clinical photographs.

Step 4: Write the Medical Case Study Report

- Follow the standard format for the report: abstract, introduction, case presentation, discussion, conclusion and references. Include additional information as outlined in the author's guideline by the journal to which you are submitting for publication.

The abstract can be written after you have completed the report, since it summarizes the entire paper.

Step 5: Submit your Medical Case Study Report to a Professional Journal

Before submitting the manuscript, you must make it clear to the editor and reviewer what your case adds to the field of medicine. In your cover letter, please consider the following:

1. Do you believe it is the first report of this kind in the literature?

2. Will it significantly advance our understanding of a particular mechanism?

3. Is it an original case report of interest to a particular clinical speciality of medicine or will it have a broader clinical impact across more than one area of medicine?

6.5 Preparation of Manuscript Sections for Case Reports

Select a proper professional journal to submit your case report and read the instruction to the author section. The journal should cover your scientific research or medical professional area. Every journal has its special format. It is wise to read the published case reports on this journal to understand better the requirements of the *instruction to authors'* section. In the following part, we will introduce the usual format of most journals.

Manuscripts for case reports submitted to medical journals should be divided into the following sections in the following order:

- Title
- Abstract
- Keywords
- Introduction
- Case presentations
- Discussion
- Conclusion
- Patient's perspective
- List of abbreviations used
- Consent
- Competing interest
- Author's contributions
- Author's information
- Acknowledgement
- Endnotes

- References
- Illustrations and figures
- Tables and caption (if any)
- Preparing additional files

Title

The first page of the manuscript should be a dedicated title page, including the article's title. The title should include the study design, i.e., a case report.

Example: An Unusual Etiology of Chronic Subdural Hematoma — Case Report

All authors' full names, institutional addresses, and email addresses must be included on the title page. The corresponding author should also be indicated.

Some journals require the title page to be submitted separately for peer-review. The editorial board will blindly and randomly choose reviewers, which will avoid the reviewers knowing the authors of the submitted manuscript.

Some journals permit the author to recommend one or two reviewers in the related scientific area if the disease or medical problems are too rare or complex for most reviewers.

The recommended reviewers should not be on the authors' list. It is better not to recommend reviewers in the same institute as the authors.

Usually, the editorial board does not invite the recommended reviewers by the authors unless the case is rare. For most of the journals, the author has the authority to refuse some reviewers to the editorial board. In the submission process, the author should list the name and institute of the refused reviewers.

That means you can avoid the reviewers you don't like. By the way, in all the review processes, the author will never know who reviewed their manuscript, whether the manuscript is accepted or rejected.

Abstract

This should start on page 2 of the manuscript. The words of the abstract must not exceed the journal requirement, usually 200 to 350 words. Do not use abbreviations or references in the abstract. The abstract should be structured into three sections and should make clear how the case report adds to the medical literature:

- Introduction

An introduction about why this case is important and needs to be reported. Please include information on whether this is the first report of this kind in the literature.

- Case presentation

Brief detail of what the patient (s) presented with, including the patient's age, sex and ethnic background.

- Conclusion

A brief conclusion of what the reader should learn from the case report and the clinical impact. Is it an original case report of interest to particular clinical impact across medicine? Please include information on how it will significantly advance our knowledge of a particular disease etiology or drug mechanism.

Keywords

There is no strict requirement as to how many keywords should be presented. Usually, there should be 3 to 6 keywords representing the main content of the article. The most important keywords should be presented or listed first. Sometimes the editorial board will invite reviewers based on the information of the keywords, which present what research area to which the case belongs.

Introduction

The introduction section should explain the background of the case, including the disorder, usual presentation and progression and the explanation of the presentation if it is a new disease. If it is a case discussing an adverse drug interaction, the introduction should give details of the drug's common use and any previously reported side effects. It should also include a brief literature review.

Case Presentations

This should present all relevant details concerning the case.

The case presentation should contain:

- A description of the patient's relevant demographic information (without adding any details that could lead to the identification of the patient).
- Any relevant medical history of the patient.
- The symptoms and signs.
- Any tests that were carried out and a description of any treatment or intervention. If it is a case series, then details must be included for all patients.

Discussion

This is an optional section for additional comments that provide relevant information not included in the case presentation and that put the case in context or explain specific treatment decisions.

Conclusion

This should state clearly the main conclusions of the case presentation and give a clear explanation of their importance and relevance. It should answer the question: is it an original case report of interest to a particular clinical specialty, or will it have a broader clinical impact across medicine? It should include information on how it will significantly advance knowledge of a particular disease etiology or drug mechanism.

Patient's Perspective

This section is an opportunity for the patient to add a description of the case from their perspective. The patient should be encouraged to state what originally made them seek medical advice, describe their symptoms, whether the symptoms were better or worse at different times, how many tests and treatments affected them, and the current status of the problem.

This section can be written as deemed appropriate by the patient; however, it should not includes identifying irrelevant information to the case reported. Consent to publish forms will be requested on submission for any manuscript that includes a patient's perspective.

List of Abbreviations Used

If abbreviations are used in the text, they should be defined in the text at first use, and a list of abbreviations can be provided, which should precede the competing interests and authors' contributions.

Consent

Manuscripts will not be peer-reviewed if a statement of patient consent is not presented.

This section is compulsory. It should provide a statement to confirm that the patient has given their informed consent to publish the case report. The editorial office may request copies of the consent documentation at any time.

We recommend the following wording is used for the consent section. *"Written informed consent was obtained from the patient for publication of this case report and accompanying images. A copy of the written consent is available for review by the editor-in- chief of this journal."*

Competing Interests

Authors are required to complete a declaration of competing interests. All competing interests that are declared will be listed at the end of the published articles. Where an author gives no competing interests, the listing will read : *"the author (s) declare (s) that they have no competing interests"*.

Authors' Contributions

To give appropriate credit to each author of a paper, the individual contributions of authors to the manuscripts should be specified in this section. We suggest the following format (please use initials to refer to each author's contribution). Criteria for authorship should include somebody who initiated the idea, designed the scientific research or medical care and follow-up, the oversight responsibility of the organization of the project and manuscript, analyzed and interpreted data, performed a special examination, and was a major contributor in writing the manuscript. All authors should read and approve the manuscripts. All contributors who do not meet the criteria for authorship should be listed in an acknowledgment section.

Acknowledgements

Please acknowledge anyone who contributed to the article by making substantial contributions to conception, design, acquisition of data, analysis and interpretation of data, or who was involved in drafting the manuscript or critically revising it for important intellectual content but does not meet the criteria for authorship. Please also include the source (s) of funding for each author and the manuscript (s) preparation.

Endnotes

Endnotes should be designated within the text using a superscript lowercase letter, and all notes (along with their corresponding letter) should be included in the endnotes section. Please format this section in a paragraph rather than a list.

References

Authors must search for and cite published case reports that are relevant to the case they are presenting. The most popular style is in following order:

- Authors
- Title of the article
- Journal
- Published year
- Volume (issue)
- Page number

Example: Turfe, Z.A., et al., Endovascular coiling versus parent artery occlusion for treatment of cavernous carotid aneurysms: a meta-analysis. Journal of Neuro-Interventional Surgery, 2015, 7 (4), p.250-255.

6.6 Preparing Illustrations and Figures

6.6.1 Figure

A figure can be defined as an illustration or explanatory diagram in a text. Read the *"instruction for authors"*, please note that some journals can only publish no more than ten figures in each case report. If you have more than ten figures and feel that all are essential for understanding the case report, please make this clear in your covering letter, explaining why the figures are necessary. Figures and tables should be sequentially referenced. Authors should include all relevant supporting data with each article. In some journals, case reports accompanied by video/images have high priority for publishing.

6.6.2 Illustration

Illustration is an example serving to clarify or prove something. The Illustration should be provided as separate files, not embedded in the text file. Each figure should include a single illustration and should fit on a single page in portrait format. If a figure consists of separate parts, a single composite illustration file must be submitted containing all parts of the figures. In some journals, there is no charge for the use of color figures. Authors should make every effort to preserve the patient's anonymity by removing or concealing any identifiable features, including birthmarks and tattoos.

Special attention should be given to the head and face images, ensuring that only the relevant features are shown. Publication of facial images will be subject to approval by the editor-in-chief.

6.6.3 Legend

Legends are captions that explain figures, tables, or images in a manuscript. The legends should be included in the main manuscript text file at the end of the document, rather than being a part of the figure file.

For each figure, the following information should be provided:
- Figure number (in sequence, using Arabic numerals, i.e., figure 1, 2, 3, etc.)
- Short title of the figure
- Detail legend

The legend should include a brief description of the exact location of images on the patient, the types of images (example: CT scan/MRI), and time about progression.

Example: one week after surgery. There must be no abbreviations unless they are expanded (excluding commonly used abbreviations). Please note that it is the responsibility of the author (s) to obtain permission from the copyright holder to reproduce figures or tables that have previously been published elsewhere.

6.7 Preparing Tables

Each table should be numbered and cited in sequence using the Arabic numerals (i.e., 1, 2, 3, etc.). Tables should also have a title (above the table) that summarizes the whole table. Detailed legends may then follow, but they should be concise. Tables should always be cited in text in consecutive numerical order.

Columns and rows of the data should be made visibly distinct. Tables should not be embedded as figures nor as a spreadsheet files. According to the journal's requirement, tabular data provided as additional files can be uploaded as an excel spreadsheet (.xs) or comma-separated values (.csv). As with all files, please use the standard files extensions.

6.8 Preparing Additional Files

Usually, case reports encourage authors to provide data sets, tables, movies, or other information as additional files. Case reports accompanied by video/movie images have high priority for publication. Additional files are published along with the article and links provided to the file as submitted by the author. A journal requires a maximum file size for additional files, and files are usually scanned on submission. Additional files can be in many formats and are downloaded from the final published article as submitted by the author.

If additional materials are provided, the following information is listed in a separate section of the manuscript text:

- File name (e.g., additional file 1)
- File format including the correct file extension

Example: .pdf, .xls, .txt, .pptx (including name and URL of an appropriate viewer if format is unusual).

- Title of the data
- Description of the data

Additional files should be named "additional file 1" and so on, and should be explicitly referenced by the file name within the body of the article, e.g., *"An additional video file shows this in more detail [see additional file 1]"*.

6.8.1 Style and Language

Submitted manuscripts must have a high standard of written English. Authors are advised to write clearly and simply and to have their article proofread by colleagues before submission. Before submission, it is better to check and correct misused words, spelling errors, missing references or incomplete citation information. Manuscripts that are poorly written or with too many mistakes are usually rejected directly or returned to the authors for revision before peer-review.

6.8.2 Language Editing

For authors who are not a native-English speakers, it is better to invite a native-English speaker with scientific expertise to edit your manuscript.

6.8.3 Abbreviation

Abbreviations should be used as sparingly as possible. They should be defined when first used, and a list of abbreviation can be provided following the main manuscript text.

6.8.4 Case Overview

Usually, authors are required to answer series of questions as part of the submission process.

6.9 Submission Process

Many journals require online submission of papers. The author should register on the required website to obtain a username and password to log in. Sometimes the website automatically offers a password; the author cannot change the password. After logging in, authors provide personal information according to the journal's requirement to create an account. When the account is successfully created, the author can submit their manuscript and upload additional files.

As part of the submission process, a series of questions can be asked that the author needs to answer before submitting the manuscript.

Outline of the case overview content usually required is given below:

Patient's Detail:

- Age
- Sex
- Country of resident

Clinical Detail:

- Reasons for case presentation
- Primary diagnosis
- Secondary diagnosis (if applicable)
- Investigations carried out before a diagnosis
- Pharmaceutical preparation
- Geographical location of this report

6.10 Writing Better Science Paper

Clarity, simplicity, and accuracy are the three most important attributes of a well-written scientific paper. Good writing always speaks for itself and does not need to be dressed up with complicated words or an incomprehensible list of acronyms. Anyone from anywhere in the world should be able to read your paper. Therefore, no matter how complex the names of chemicals, species or analytical techniques might be, explaining the underlying concepts of your research in simple language is a definite advantage for you and the community.

This section helps to identify easy steps that you can take to improve your writing skills and the outcome of the publication process.

From the time you developed the idea to write a case report, there will be countless opportunities to simplify, clarify, and get people as excited about your medical work as you are. You will find out how descriptive titles, concise abstracts, uncluttered graphics, and simple language can all play a vital part in opening up all the amazing developments that happen in science to a wide audience, as well as making editors, referees, and readers sit up and take notice of your work.

6.10.1 Title

The title of a paper is important because it is one of the first things that an editor/

reviewer/reader sees when they look at your manuscript. Therefore, it is important to grab their attention right away and give them an idea of why your paper is a scientific breakthrough. Be specific, not too technical and concise.

The other thing to consider is that internet and scientific search tools often search by manuscript title, so getting your paper read and cited is important to get some of the key aspects of the research into the title. A good tip is to think which search terms you would use to find your paper through a web search.

For a basic example, consider a manuscript entitled *"Effect of Chinese herbs on the patients with Parkinson's disease"*.

What is the effect? Which type of Chinese herbs? What stage of the disease? The title looks like a review, not a case report of scientific research. The editor/reviewer/ reader gets nothing but questions out of the title. Much better might be: *"Effect of XYZ herbs on the motor function with Parkinson's disease patients: case series."*

The editor/reviewer/reader immediately knows what the paper is about and will want to read more.

Finally, avoid adding every detail from the paper into the title — the title should not be confused with or replace an abstract. The most read and most cited articles often have a short and simple title.

6.10.2 Abstract

Imagine you have twenty seconds to explain the project you have been working on for months or years to another scientist who is not familiar with your area of research.

You would probably tell them the one or two main outcomes without going into excessive technical detail. This is a good way to think about writing your abstract. A good abstract is concise, explains the main findings of the research, but does not overwhelm the reader with technicalities. You want the reader to be interested enough to read the whole paper to find the technical details themselves. Good abstract writing is a key skill for scientists, as it is necessary for the conference, grant proposal, and job interviews, so take your time and think about making an impact.

6.10.3 Introduction

The introduction is a little different from the short abstract. The reader needs to know the background to your research and, most importantly, why your research is important in this context. What critical question does your research address? Why should the reader be interested? Setting the scene well for your reader is vital to know the importance of your research.

However, try to avoid making too bold claims, like *"this is a potential cure for all cancers"* (unless it is, then you really can shout about it). Do not forget that the first impressions of the editor and reviewers when they first read your manuscript are important too, so if you can convey why your project is so exciting to them, this can only be a good thing!

6.10.4 Method and Material/Experimental

Possibly the easiest section of the whole manuscript to write — write down what you did, how much you used and how long. Easy though it may be to write, there are still things you can do to make your experimental section an easy read.

Don't forget, this is the evidence for all of your ideas presented in the paper, and some people will use or try to reproduce your methods. Therefore, clarity and good presentation help.

6.10.5 Results and Discussion

After so many months on your project and achieved some great results, it is time for presenting them in a paper. Now, if you want to bore your reader (s), tell them about all the hours you have spent testing every solvent, catalyst, and additive you could think of and all the trouble you have had with the HPLC (high-performance liquid chromatography). So, the best advice is to keep your focus and make your result and discussion concise but informative.

Sometimes, the most interesting and discussible parts of research are the anomalies or the things that don't make sense. Don't ignore these outliers because referees will likely ask you to comment on your strange results. Discussion of strange results is often as valuable as focusing on the expected findings. It can help understand the more subtle features of a reaction, a catalyst, or a material. And who knows, your one weird result might be enough to open up a whole new area of research.

6.10.6 Graphics and Tables

Graphics are the most eye-catching part of scientific papers.

Simplicity is the key with graphics. Try to avoid clutter and putting too much text in a graphic. A good graphic can get its message across to the reader without the need for lots of explanatory text, so if you find you are putting a lot of text in, you may need to change your graphic. Getting your graphics right helps towards faster publication and clearer understanding.

6.10.7 Conclusion

The conclusion should contain a little more about the results, what can be learned, and some speculation about the implications.

6.10.8 References

Like the experimental section, the reference section is very easy to write, but you can do some small things to make it user-friendly. Especially when referencing the introduction of your manuscript, a good tip is only to reference the most relevant papers or some good thorough reviews on your particular area of research.

Perhaps you might not think about it, but this shows the editor and the reviewers that you know your field well and understand what is important in this context.

6.10.9 Cover Letter

Often overlooked in submissions, your cover letter is your chance to talk directly to the editor and highlight all the most important results of your research. It can either make a great first impression or leave the editor uninspired, so it is a fantastic opportunity to make the editor sit up and take notice of your paper.

Much like an introduction, a good cover letter explains to the editor the critical question your research addresses, how you have answered this question, and why it is significant to the wider community.

The best cover letters are concise and clearly explain the advances and discoveries made in the research. Remember, journals receive many papers per day and editors see hundreds of manuscripts per year, so take every opportunity you can to get your work noticed.

Presentation at Academic Conference

7.1 Information Box

When an author presents the slides of a presentation, they follow several procedures. These procedures help the authors to express their idea easily. A set of slides should provide the audience with the author's idea and conclusion.

First, have a clear and simple structure. To organize a set of slides for a scientific presentation, your presentation's structure should be as follows: aims and background (descriptions and goals), methods, results and conclusion (implications and limitations).

Next, the slides should describe in detail and highlight the main purpose. That is, the presenter should summarize the slides into several conclusions. Discussion should be around, or to prove these conclusions.

Finally, several little tips may make the slides more attractive and efficient. In a set of slides, photos and other images should be used to enhance the presentation. At least one picture should be used on almost every slide. Do not use lots of text, and words should be in a large, clear-to-read font. Interesting charts and graphs also need to enhance a presentation. These graphs need to be easy to follow, and the colors should be conservative and no more than three colors in one slide.

7.2 Grammar Tip: Syntax

You need to understand two important elements of effective English language communication: *syntax* and *diction*. Syntax is the arrangement of words that make a sentence; diction is the choice of words. We will discuss in this chapter the first of the two: Syntax!

> *The patient rested peacefully.*
> *The doctors operated quickly.*
> *The medicine worked well.*

Although each of the above is a different subject sentence, the syntax is identical; this is called "parallelism" and is very important for effective communication; particularly writing.

Parallel structure is important when you show that several details in a sentence or paragraph (or talk) are equally important. Look at this example:

The patient chose to have a consultation, and then let a doctor examine her.

Now this:

The patient chose to have a consultation, and an examination by a doctor.

The second example is parallel as the syntax is the same throughout the sentence; the first example is not parallel.

A common mistake made by Chinese when writing English is to mixed tenses; look at this example:

The patient will do well after the operation and is recovering quickly.

In this example the paralelism is lost because the sentence starts with future tense (will…) and ends with present tense (recove<u>ring</u>…).

The parallel version is:

The patient will do well after the operation and will recover quickly.

Remember: check that you maintain the same syntax and tense throughout a sentence. Next chapter we will discuss diction.

7.3 Cross-Cultural Awareness

A common complaint made by foreigners (westerners) in China is the difficulty in telling doctors and pharmacists that they want western medicine, not Chinese medicine; also, they question why they can not buy medium-strength pain killers (aspirin and paracetamol) in many drug stores. Foreigners are interested in immediate relief, hence their preference for fast-acting western medications. Foreign patients are also more likely to question a doctor's prescription and want detailed information about the pharmaceuticals; if the medicine is unfamiliar, they may ask for scientific evidence of its efficacy.

Should an occasion arise where your patient is questioning your prescription, do not take it personally; it is common practice in most western patient-doctor interactions.

7.4 Presentations: Academic Conference/Seminar

Many times we are aware of our poor performance, but we find excuses instead of improvement. *We should not take pride* in the level of the disaster of our presentation and expect others to understand in the knowledge that they, too, have been in a similar situation.

7.4.1 Typical Mistakes

Typical mistakes that presenters know that they make and continue to make them anyway:

- No clear structure / no clear message
- No eye contact with the audience
- Too much text — hard to find key info
- No images
- Presenter reads the text on the slides — word for word
- Monotone voice + no enthusiasm
- Too long + too many technical details
- Too much animation
- Too small fonts + bad use of color
- No match between what the presenter says and what appears on the slides

Other Key Problems Are:

- The final slide has no call to action.
- The presenter spent too much time preparing the slides but no time to practice them.

7.4.2 Solution

Before you start preparing your presentation, you need to think deeply about the following:

1. Why did you choose your specific research topic?

Simply saying that "my professor told me to study it", or "I like the topic" is not enough. It would be best if you looked inside yourself. Go back into your past; where was the seed sown?

2. Why is your research important to you, and why should it be important also for your audience and society in general?

If you can't think of reasons for this, you will never give a convincing presentation.

3. Why is it important to tell other people about it?

Think in terms not only of the benefits but also what would happen if your research was NOT carried out.

When you have thought about these questions, then:

- Think about a captivating way to introduce your research in the first few slides.

- Give your audience a clear plan (you can do this orally; you don't necessarily need a slide).
- Structure your presentation as follows: description of problem + goals; method; results; implications and limitations.
- Be concise. Only put essential information on your slides.

IMPACT:

If you manage to put all the above into practice, you will be making a start to becoming a passionate, convincing, interesting, enthusiastic and confident presenter. This will hopefully gain you respect and credibility; people will want to contact you, people will want to work with you, and your publications will be read.

7.5 Project Proposal

7.5.1 Typical Mistake

One of the most serious mistakes you can make when writing a proposal is not to think about the reviewer, who has to read it and judge whether it is worthy of funding. Understanding the reviewer's work helps to have a clear idea of the review process. The stages listed below have been simplified and are certainly not universal — every review board will have its procedure.

Review Process:

Stage 1: Each reviewer is given up to 15 proposals. Of these 15, they must choose one or two to "defend" at the final review meeting. First, the reviewers very quickly screen the proposals and eliminate as many proposals as they can.

Stage 2: If the reviewer had 15 proposals in stage 1, by stage 2, they have probably narrowed this number down to a shortlist of 5 or 6. They will opt for those proposals that are laid out and which have clear aims and benefits. The reviewer then selects those proposals that they feel are the most pertinent to the call for proposals and then makes a more detailed analysis.

Stage 3: The reviewer chooses 1 or 2 proposals to defend/support/promote at the review meeting. They make a very detailed analysis of why the proposal should be funded.

Stage 4: At the review meeting, the reviewer tries to convince the board that your proposal is the best and will try to find faults in the proposals chosen by the other reviewers.

7.5.2 Solution

Reviewers invest a lot of time in stage 3. Your proposal must be worthy of such a time investment. Most researchers focus on the following:

- Subject/topic
- Background
- Aims
- Design
- Time frame
- Cost
- Partners involved and level of experience

However, the reviewers are probably asking themselves different questions: is the project of the moment? Is it a problem that needs solving? What does it add to the state of the art? Is it original and innovative? How multi-disciplinary is it?

Other questions that you need to answer are:

- How clear are your objectives? (if the reviewers can't understand your aims, they will stop reading your proposal)
- How feasible and credible are they?
- How appropriate is the methodology/approach?
- How realistic are the milestones?
- How realistic is the cost?
- Would the potential results justify such a cost?
- How have the possible results been presented/highlighted?
- How can these results be exploited in other fields?

Think about the reviewer — constantly! Try at all times to minimize the reviewer's time and effort in reading your proposal. Think about how you can facilitate their work by:

- Making the reading experience as enjoyable as possible (this doesn't mean they have to be entertained, but where you can be concise, be concise).
- Using a clear layout that helps the reviewer to focus on what is important.
- Providing the reviewer with the weapons (i.e., the added value of your project) they need to win the battle for funds against the competing projects.

IMPACT:

If you make your proposal as clear and readable as possible, you will massively enhance your chances of your proposal being chosen by a reviewer. Also, never forget the big picture. Sometimes it can be the big picture that gives meaning to a project or the results of a study. Try always to think outside your academic box!

Many extremely well-presented proposals written with the reviewer in mind have likely been allocated funds even though there may have been more worthy projects presented poorly in their proposals.

8.1 Information Box

Hospitals vary widely in the services they offer and, therefore, in the departments they have. Hospitals may have acute services such as an emergency department or specialist trauma center, burn unit, surgery, or urgent care. These may then be backed up by more specialist units such as cardiology or coronary care unit (CCU), intensive care unit (ICU), neurology, cancer center, and obstetrics and gynecology.

Some hospitals will also have outpatient departments, while others may have chronic treatment units such as behavioral health services, dentistry, dermatology, psychiatric ward, rehabilitation services (Rehab), and physical therapy.

Common hospital support units include a dispensary or pharmacy, pathology, and radiology. On the non-medical side, there often are medical records departments and/or a release of information department. Nursing services are considered one of the most important aspects in the process of distinguished medical care.

8.2 Grammar Tip: Diction

In the last chapter, we discussed the first of two important English communication skills — syntax; now, we will discuss the second — diction! Diction is the choice of words used.

Although many Chinese doctors are familiar with English medical terms, their choice of the words surrounding their medical terms often do not equate to the quality of their professional vocabulary; indeed, many of what we may call *"functional vocabulary"* are little advanced from what they learned in primary and middle school. Space does not allow us to go into too much detail on this topic, so we will provide you with some simple techniques to mature your functional vocabulary.

The most important parts of speech in English are verbs and nouns. A simple method to elevate your vocabulary from mundane to power-vocabulary is to count the syllables in the verbs and nouns you utilize. Syllables are the group of letters that produce a sound and, when combined form a word; for example, the word *"medicine"* has three syllables — *me/di/cine.*

NOTE: Every syllable must contain a vowel **sound** (a,e, i,o,u).

Power vocabulary is the words that contain two or more syllables. Look at this simple sentence:

The nurse quickly opened the door and went out of the ward.

The nurse exited the ward hurriedly. (Powerful)

The doctor told the patient what he would do.

The doctor advised the patient of the treatment. (Powerful)

Count the syllables in your verbs and nouns; if they have only one, change the word to a polysyllabic word. If you look up a thesaurus *(a dictionary for synonyms-different words with the same meaning),* you are sure to find power words. Most modern computers have a thesaurus built-in; put the cursor on the word, right-click your mouse, and a drop-menu should appear showing "synonyms", click on this, and you may find the power-word you seek.

And know that in English, the less you say, the better, so use power vocabulary to get your information across.

8.3 Cross-Cultural Awareness

I overheard a foreign woman talking to a friend on her phone when I was recently in a cafe. "*The office looked like a white broom closet with a desk and chair in it.*" The "*office*" she was referring to was a doctor's room in a Chinese hospital. Rightly or wrongly, many foreigners develop their confidence in professionals based on body language and environment; the "environment" is the subject of this article.

Western doctors' offices are relatively large and comfortable, even in hospitals; indeed, many have an examination room attached to the office proper. A western doctor's medical environment provides an air of confidence that patients positively respond to.

So, when a foreigner has to visit a Chinese doctor in a hospital, they are often taken aback by the spartan nature of the examination environment, they find it difficult to have confidence in the doctor and, therefore, the prognosis; this negativity is exacerbated with other patients wandering in and out.

I understand it is little; if anything, you can do about the environment you consult in, be aware that if a foreign patient looks bewildered, it is because the whole Chinese medical landscape is foreign to them…you will have to apply your best people skills to relieve their consternation.

8.4 Locations in the Hospital

No.	Rooms and departments in hospitals and clinics	
1	Accident and emergency (A&E)	The accident and emergency department of a hospital
2	Admissions	The part of the hospital where patients are required to provide personal information and sign consent forms before being taken to the hospital unit or ward. If the individual is critically ill, then, this information is usually obtained from a family member
3	Anesthetics room/department	Doctors in this department give anesthetic for operations and procedures
4	On-call room	A room in a hospital intended for doctors/staff to rest in while they are on call or due to be
5	Casualty/trauma center	The part of the hospital where people go when they are injured or suddenly become ill. The official name for this is accident and emergency (A&E). The American word is the emergency room
6	Central sterile service department (CSSD)/sterile processing department (SPD)/central supply department (CSD)	A place in a hospital and other health care facilities that perform sterilization and other actions on medical equipment, devices, and consumables
7	Consulting room	A room where a doctor examines a patient and discuss their medical problems with them
8	Coronary care unit (CCU)/cardiac intensive care unit (CICU)	A hospital ward specialized in the care of patients with cardiac conditions that require continuous monitoring and treatment
9	Day room	A room in the hospital where patients can go during the day to watch television, read or talk
10	Delivery room	A room in a hospital where women give birth
11	Dispensary	A place in a hospital where you can get medicines and drugs
12	Diagnostic imaging	Also known as the X-ray department and/or radiology department
13	Emergency department	The part of the hospital where people go when they are injured or suddenly become ill

continued

No.	Rooms and departments in hospitals and clinics	
14	Emergency room (ER)	The A&E in the hospital
15	High dependency unit (HDU)	The department of a hospital for people who are very ill or badly injured, but need less care than people in the intensive care
16	Housekeeping	The department of a hospital that is responsible for cleaning rooms
17	Intensive care /critical care	The department of a hospital for people who are so ill or badly injured that they need to have special medical care and be watched closely
18	Maternity ward	The part of a hospital where pregnant women or women who have just given birth to babies are looked after
19	Nursery	An area in a hospital where new babies are looked after until they go home
20	Nurses' station /nursing station	An area in the hospital where nurses and other health care staff work behind when not working directly with patients and where they perform some of their duties
21	Operating room	An operating theatre
22	Operating theatre	A room in a hospital where doctors perform medical operations
23	Outpatient department (OPD)/ outpatient clinic	The part of a hospital designed for the treatment of people with health problems who visit the hospital for diagnosis or treatment, but do not at this time require to be admitted for a an overnight care
24	Padded cell	A room in a hospital for mentally ill people, with soft material on the walls so that they cannot hurt themselves
25	Pharmacy	The part of a hospital where medicines are prepared
26	Sickroom/short stay unit (SSU)	A room where someone who is ill rests or gets medical treatment usually up to 23 hours
27	Surgery	A room in a hospital where doctors do surgery
28	Theatre	A room in a hospital used for medical operations. The American word is operating room

continued

No.	Rooms and departments in hospitals and clinics	
29	Unit	A department of an institution, especially a section in the hospital that has a particular purpose
30	Ward	A large room in a hospital with beds for people to stay

8.5 Professional Titles

There are multiple levels of practicing medicine. Many people exist on a physician team, each having their responsibilities. Some are licensed to practice medicine, while others are studying hard to get there. The typical medical hierarchy of top heads at hospitals and the general responsibilities of each role from the top down is shown below:

No.	Professional title	General responsibilities
1	Medical director	The medical director of a hospital is an industry leader in charge of overseeing every single physician on the staff
2	Head of department	When you work at a hospital, the doctor responsible for a patient's treatment plan is the attending. There may be times when your attending is too busy or preoccupied to answer your questions. In that case, you need the head of the department associated with the issue
3	Attending physician	The senior doctors in a hospital are the attending physicians. They are responsible for the major decision-making related to a patient's treatment
4	Fellow	Right below the attending physicians when it comes to responsibilities are fellows. After completing their primary residencies, these doctors work on fellowship or advanced training in a special medical specialty
5	Residents	Residents are doctors working in a hospital that have already graduated from medical school. They have also taken and passed the required national licensing exams. Each resident is licensed to practice medicine as an medical doctor (MD). However, this person must have supervision when working with patients until three years of hand's training are completed

continued

No.	Professional title	General responsibilities
6	Chief resident	This person works at the highest senior level for all residents. The chief resident is in charge of directing activities of all other residents at the hospital
7	Senior resident	Immediately below the chief is the senior resident. Generally, this doctor is in the third year of residency, depending on the specialty
8	Junior resident	Just below the seniors are the junior residents. These doctors are generally in the second years of their residency
9	Intern	Once a medical student has graduated from medical school and started practicing medicine under supervision, this doctor is called an intern. At some hospital, they are referred to as first year residents if they have started residency Although interns do have medical degrees and are referred to as doctor, they are not licensed to practice medicine without supervision. They must be supervised by senior residents or senior MDs when working with patients
10	Medical student	When a person is studying to become a doctor in medical school, that person is called a medical student. This person hasn't graduated and doesn't have a medical degree yet

Other Clinical and Non-Clinical Professional Titles

Clinical

No.	Professional title	General responsibilities
1	Medical technologist	A medical technologist works in a hospital's lab to perform tests, they prepare blood, tissue and other samples and use specialized equipment to test them
2	Radiologist/radiologic technician	Radiologic technicians perform X-rays to help doctors produce diagnostic images for their patients
3	Dietician	Dieticians educate patients on proper diet and help them manage conditions, such as obesity and diabetes
4	Respiratory therapist	Respiratory therapists treat patients who have difficulty breathing. They also work with devices like ventilators and artificial airways
5	Registered nurses	Nurses support doctors by caring for sick, injured or recovering patients and communicating with patients and families

continued

Clinical

No.	Professional title	General responsibilities
6	Occupational therapist	Occupational therapists help sick, disabled, injured and recovering patients perform daily tasks, such as dressing, bathing and preparing meals
7	Pharmacist	Pharmacists are health professionals who specialized in the use of medicines, as they deal with the composition, effects, mechanism of action and proper and effective use of drugs
8	Physician assistant	Physician assistants assess, diagnose and treat patients under a licensed physician's supervision
9	Surgeon	The surgeon operates on patients to repair injuries or help treat diseases or conditions. They generally specialize in one type of surgery, such as general surgery, orthopedic, pediatric surgery, plastic surgery, neurosurgery, etc.
10	Anesthesiologist	Anesthesiologists give patients medications that remove pain and sensation during surgery

Non-clinical

No.	Professional title	General responsibilities
11	Medical admission clerk	Admission clerks greet patients entering the hospital and gather their medical and personal information and reason for visiting
12	Medical record clerk	Medical record clerks organize and file patient information, such as medical histories, and admission and discharge documents
13	Coding specialist	Coding specialists work in the billing department. They classify and code health care claims so the hospital can receive payment from insurance companies and health care programs
14	Medical social worker	Social workers help patients and their families deal with the physical, emotional and financial stress of hospitalization. They also teach nurses and doctors how to handle patients with issues like depression or anxiety
15	Information technology specialist	Information technology specialist maintain the hospital's computers, networks and servers. They keep software up to date and make sure the crucial data in the hospital computer systems is private and protected from cyber threats

continued

Non-clinical

No.	Professional title	General responsibilities
16	Human resource manager	Human resources managers oversee all hospital employee and personnel needs. They recruit, hire and train new employees and communicate with existing staff to resolve conflicts and enforce workplace policies
17	Chief executive officer	Chief executive officers are the top administrators in a hospital. They oversee the organization's daily operations as well as create long-term strategies to keep business running smoothly

8.6 Basic Neurosurgical Equipment

Most operating rooms have a basic set of equipment and areas where the different operating room staff members complete their intended tasks before, during, and after every surgical procedure.

Most neurosurgical procedures in the operating room or "theatre" involve a team of people with defined roles to meet every need encountered during the procedure. Most operating room staff include a circulating nurse, a surgical technician or nurse, an anesthesia team (some with neuro anesthesia specialists) and finally, the surgical team itself, which may have several members, such as neurosurgery attending (s), residents, medical students, fellows, etc..

8.6.1 Operating Room Setup

The diagrams below do not cover every acceptable or conceivable variation. They are meant as suggestions and as a guide to teach how the operating room can be arranged to maximize efficiency. Both right- and left-handed setups are represented for general cranial, general spinal and endonasal/transsphenoidal cases. More specific arrangements for specialized neurosurgical procedures are not covered but can be gleaned from the principles illustrated by the diagrams.

Operating Room Setup Legend (Figure 8.1-8.8)

A–anesthesia	Ae–anesthesia equipment
C–accessory equipment	I–surgical instruments
M–microscope	S–neurosurgeon
s–assistant neurosurgeon	Sn–scrub nurse or tech

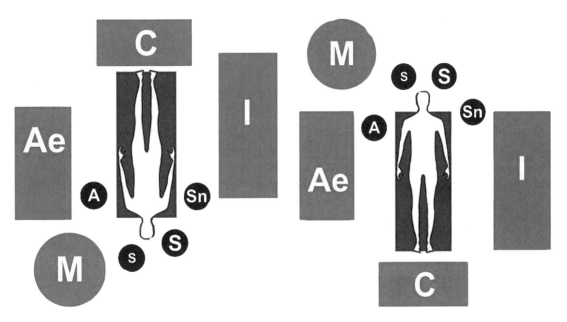

Figure 8.1 **General right-handed surgeon supine or posterior fossa craniotomy setup (cranial approach)**

Figure 8.2 **General left-handed surgeon supine or posterior fossa craniotomy setup (cranial approach)**

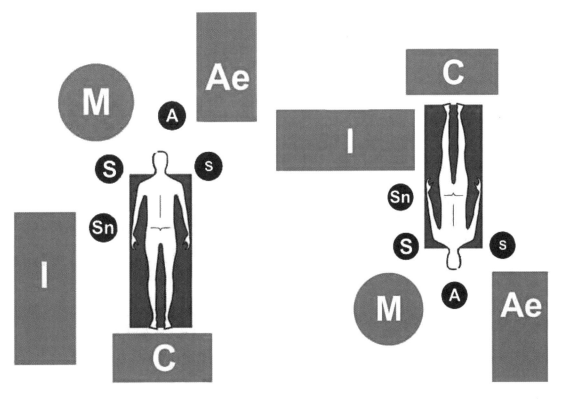

Figure 8.3 **General right-handed surgeon posterior fossa craniotomy setup (caudal approach)**

Figure 8.4 **General left-handed surgeon posterior fossa craniotomy setup (caudal approach)**

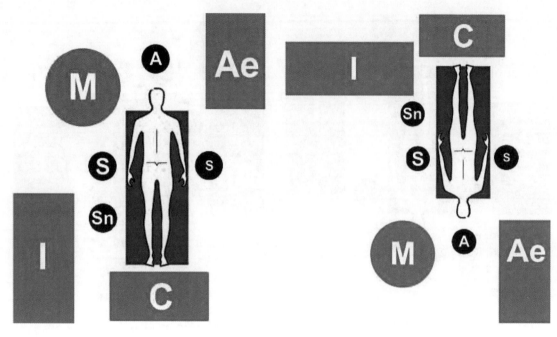

Figure 8.5 General right-handed surgeon spine procedure setup

Figure 8.6 General left-handed surgeon spine procedure setup

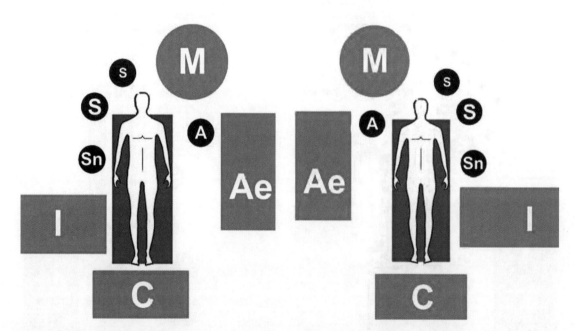

Figure 8. 7 General right-handed surgeon endonasal/transsphenoidal setup

Figure 8.8 General left-handed surgeon endonasal/transsphenoidal setup

8.6.2 Operating Room Equipment

No.	Operating room equipment
1	Operating room table
2	Mayfield head holder
3	Horseshoe
4	Greenberg retractor system: ➢ Leyla-Yagarsil retractor system ➢ Budde halo
5	Accessory equipment: ➢ Power sources for electrocautery devices ➢ Electric drill and other equipment
6	Overhead operating room light
7	Operating microscope

8.6.3 Basic Neurosurgical Trays

Despite the vast array of neurosurgical procedures performed from head to toe, most neurosurgical procedures can be done using basic instrument sets, which may be somewhat tailored to the procedure. The three most common neurosurgical instrument sets are cranial, spine, and transsphenoidal.

8.6.3.1 Basic Cranial or Trauma Instrument Set

No.	Instrument
1	**Scissors:** Adson ganglion 6¼" Malis neurological 7" curved Mayo 6¾" curved beveled Metzenbaum 7" curved Potts-DeMartel 7¼" 45° Shark edge Mayo-Stille 6¾" straight
2	**Needle holders:** Mayo-Hegar 6" heavy Ryder 6" X-Del Ryder 7" X-Del
3	**Clamps:** Allis 6" straight Foerster sponge stick 9½" straight Halstead mosquito 5" straight

continued

No.	Instrument
3	Kelly 5½" curved
	Kocher 6" straight
	Rochester-Pean 7¼" curved
4	**Dissectors/hooks:**
	Dandy nerve hook 9" straight
	Frazier dura hook 5¼"
	Joseph double hook 6½"
	Penfield 1-4
	Woodson dural separator 7"
5	**Elevators:**
	Langenbeck 7½" 16 mm
	Quervain 7¾" 6 mm
6	**Knife handles:**
	#3 with ruler
	#7 without ruler
7	**Forceps:**
	Adson 4¾" with teeth Gerald 7" with teeth Gruenwald Bayo 8"
	Tissue 5¾" straight with teeth
	Yasargil rumor 8¾"
8	**Suction tips:**
	Poppen 5½" angled 7 Fr, 9–12 Fr (Frazier)
	Dental irrigator
9	**Miscellaneous:**
	Army-Navy retractor
	Backhaus towel clips 5¼", 3½"
	Beyer rongeur 7" curved double action 4.5 mm ×19 mm (Ruskin)
	Cushing retractor 8⅜"
	Fish hooks with Songer cable
	Freiburg spatula 8" mall flat 7/8, 10/11, 13/14, 16/17 mm
	Gelpi retractor 7¼"
	Hemoclip applier traditional 8" curved, medium
	Hemoclip applier traditional 6" curved, small
	Kerrison rongeur 2-3 mm
	Leksell-Stille rongeur 9½" angled double-action 7.5 mm ×22 mm
	Mastoid retractor 7⅞"
	4×4 Prong sharp Raney appliers
	Screwdriver with blades
	Spinal fusion curette 6¾" angled
	Stille rongeur 9¼" double action (duckbill)
	Volkmann bone curette 6¾" 3.6 mm
	Weitlaner retractor 6½" blunt 3×4

8.6.3.2 Basic Spinal Instrument Set

No.	Instrument
1	**Scissors**
2	**Needle holders**
3	**Clamps**
4	**Forceps**
5	**Knife handles**
6	**Dissectors**
7	**Suction:** Frazier 7Fr, 9Fr, 12Fr
8	**Curettes:** Spinal fusion 9" straight (multiple sizes) Spinal fusion 9" angled (multiple sizes)
9	**Retractors:** Army-Navy Collis-Taylor 7¼" 76 mm Collis-Taylor 7¼" 64 mm Gelpi 7½" Love nerve root 8¼", angled 90° Weitlaner 6½" 3×4 sharp
10	**Miscellaneous:** Backhaus towel clip 5¼" Backhaus towel clip 3½" Cobb spinal elevator ⅜", ½", ¾" Langenbeck periosteal elevators Leksell rongeur 9" wide 8 mm Leksell rongeur 8½" full curved 8 mm×16 mm Dental irrigators

8.6.3.3 Basic Transsphenoidal Instrument Set

No.	Instrument
1	**Retractors**
2	**Clamps**
3	**Needle holders**
4	**Scissors**
5	**Forceps**

continued

No.	Instrument
6	**Knives and handles:** #7 knife handles #3 knife handle with ruler Sickle knife 7½" straight sharp tip adult Freer knife 6" round Ballenger swivel knife 7½" straight 4 mm
7	**Rongeurs:** Kerrison 7" 40°, 45°, 90° thin foot 1–3 mm, 2–3 mm Decker micro 6" 2 mm×6 mm Beyer rongeur 7" curved double action 4.5 mm×19 mm (Ruskin) Ostrum Antrum straight Blakesley Wilde Rhinoforce 45° Yasargil pituitary 7½" straight 3.5 mm Oldberg pituitary 7" straight 7
8	**Miscellaneous:** Poppen (Frazier) suction 5-11 Fr Dental irrigator Foerster sponge stick 9¾" straight Converse osteotome 7" straight 4 mm,6 mm, 8 mm Cottle elevatotr Boles elevator 7" blunt Fomon retractor ball Joseph skin hook 6½" single, double prong Freer elevator 7½" 4.5 mm Gorney septum elevator suction Maxillary ostium seeker 7½"

8.6.4 Basic Neurological Instrumentation

No.	General instrument	Photo
1	**Brain needle**	

continued

No.	General instrument	Photo
2	**Cotton patty**	
3	**Cotton sponge/gauge**	
4	**Suction**	
5	**Clip applier**	
6	**Irrigator**	

continued

No.	General instrument	Photo
7	**Shunt passers**	
8	**Blade/Skin knife**	
9	**Knife handle**	
10	**Monopolar**	
11	**Scissors**	

continued

No.	General instrument	Photo
12	**Suture needle**	
13	**Needle holder**	
14	**Forcep**	
15	**Bipolar forcep**	
16	**Clamp (Allis clamp)**	

continued

No.	General instrument	Photo
17	Retractor (Army-Navy retractor)	
18	Fish hook	
19	Penfield#2 (dissector)	
20	Boles elevator/periosteal	
21	Drill handle attachments	

continued

No.	General instrument	Photo
22	**Perforator drill bit/burr hole bit**	
23	**Craniotome bit**	
24	**Bone rongeur**	
25	**Kerrison rongeur**	
26	**Curette**	

continued

No.	General instrument	Photo
27	Cranial plates/fixation plates	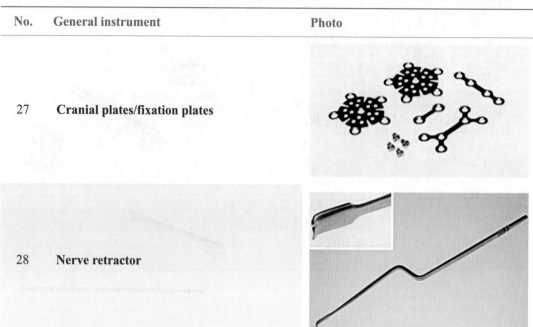
28	Nerve retractor	

8.6.5 Suture Threads

The suture threads help in holding body tissues together after surgery or an injury. It involves the use of a needle along with the thread attached to it. The suture material is categorized as either absorbable or non-absorbable. Enzymes in the body tissues can naturally digest the absorbable suture, while non-absorbable sutures are usually removed after a period.

Classification of Sutures

Degradation by organism	Absorbable Non-absorbable
Material of origin	Organic Synthetic Mineral
Quantity of filaments	Monofilament Multifilament

Catgut Suture

A catgut suture is a natural, monofilament absorbable suture that has good tensile strength. It completely disappears between 60 to 120 days.

Nylon

It's a synthetic monofilament with a smooth surface; it has offered high tension and resistance with low tissue reaction.

Polydioxanone Sutures

A type of synthetic monofilament suture, the polydioxanone suture or is used to repair various kinds of soft-tissue wounds.

Poliglecaprone Sutures

The poliglecaprone suture is a synthetic monofilament suture, generally used to repair soft tissues and vascular anastomosis procedures. These sutures promote scar-free, aesthetic healing. The suture material is used in the case of vascular anastomosis procedures that connect blood vessels.

Polyglactin Sutures

The polyglactin suture comprises a synthetic braid, which is good to repair lacerations on the face and hands and is the most preferred option for general soft tissue approximation. Polyglactin sutures typically have a mild tissue reaction for the duration of the absorption process. Still, they are a better alternative to catgut sutures as the absorption level of this suture is more predictable. Also, this suture exhibits little to no tissue reaction.

Classification of Sutures

Suture	Degradation	Origin	Quantity of filaments	Tension	Inflammatory reaction
Fast absorbing gut	Absorbable	Animal	Multifilament	Short duration	Intense
Chromic gut	Absorbable	Animal	Multifilament	Short duration	Medium
Silk	Non-absorbable	Animal	Multifilament	Medium duration	Medium
Nylon	Non-absorbable	Synthetic	Monofilament	Medium duration	Minimum
Polyglactin	Absorbable	Synthetic	Multifilament	Short duration	Minimum
Poliglecaprone	Absorbable	Synthetic	Monofilament	Long duration	Minimum
Polydioxanone	Absorbable	Synthetic	Monofilament	Not defined	Long duration
Polypropylene	Non-absorbable	Synthetic	Monofilament	Long duration	Long duration

8.7 Basic Neurosurgical Procedures and Approaches

8.7.1 Basic Neurosurgical Procedures

Neurosurgery or neurosurgical surgery is a medical specialty associated with preventing and treating various disorders related to the nervous system, including the brain, spinal cord, peripheral nerve, et c.. Trained and expert neurosurgeons perform these neurosurgical procedures. Here are some of the most common types of neurosurgical procedures performed by a neurosurgeon.

1. Brain surgery

(1) Craniotomy and craniectomy

A Craniotomy is one of the procedures where a portion of a patient's skull is removed. A **craniotomy** may be done to remove a brain tumor or abnormal brain tissue; on the other hand, a **craniectomy** is a neurosurgical procedure in which part of the skull is removed to allow a swelling brain room to expand without being squeezed. It is performed on victims of traumatic brain injury, stroke, Chiari malformation, and other conditions associated with raised intracranial pressure. **(Figure 8.9)**

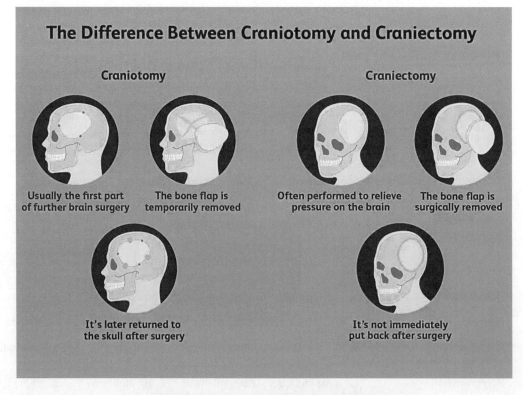

Figure 8.9 **Craniotomy and craniectomy**

(2) External ventricular drain (EVD)/ventriculostomy

The external ventricular drain (EVD) is one of the most basic and essential procedures that a junior resident must master. Still, even the most experienced can face difficulties if the technical principles are not respected. This technique is lifesaving for patients suffering from life-threatening hydrocephalus and intraventricular hemorrhage. EVD is also known as ventriculostomy, a procedure in which a doctor will use a tube to remove excess fluid in a patient's brain. This is a procedure performed without implantation.

EVD procedure steps (Figure 8.10):

- Instill local anesthesia.
- Make linear incision down to bone and scrape periosteum.
- Penetrate cranium with twist drill in the trajectory determined for ventricular cannulation and pierce pia and dura with scalpel.
- Prime ventricular catheter.

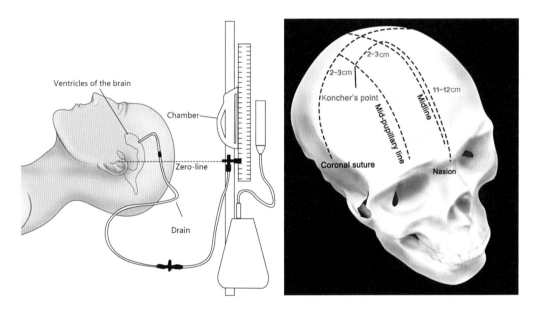

Figure 8.10 **External ventricular drain (EVD)**

(3) Ventriculoperitoneal shunt (VPS)

This is also a procedure used to remove the increasing build-up of fluid in someone's brain. In this case, a shunt is implanted into the brain to drain the excess fluid accumulated in the head. **(Figure 8.11)**

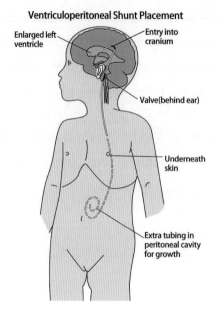

Figure 8.11 **Ventriculoperitoneal shunt (VPS)**

2. Spine surgery

(1) Discectomy and microdiscectomy

Pain radiating due to herniated discs can be practically unbearable. These disc problems can be fixed with surgery in most cases. **Discectomy** is a common procedure that involves removing the damaged disc. **Microdiscectomy** is a neurosurgical procedure used to treat people suffering from painful herniated discs in the lumbar area. **(Figure 8.12)**

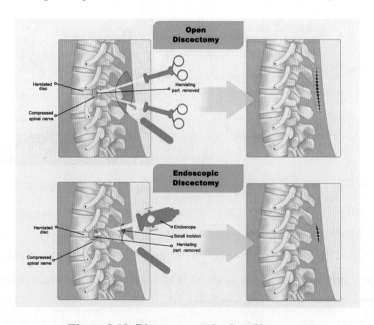

Figure 8.12 **Disectomy and microdisectomy**

(2) Laminotomy and laminectomy

Laminotomy is a minimally invasive procedure where small incisions are made in the skin during the surgery to remove a small portion of the lamina or vertebral bone. This is a common procedure for patients who are suffering from severe back pain. **Laminectomy** is a surgical procedure to remove the back of one or more vertebrae, usually to give access to the spinal cord or to relieve pressure on nerves. **(Figure 8.13)**

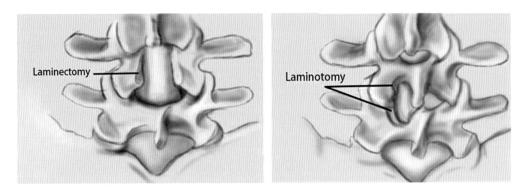

Figure 8.13   **Laminotomy and laminectomy**

(3) Spinal fusion

This procedure is used to treat degenerative diseases or traumatic injuries of the spine. A spinal fusion surgical procedure is performed to keep the patient's spine in a stable position. **(Figure 8.14)**

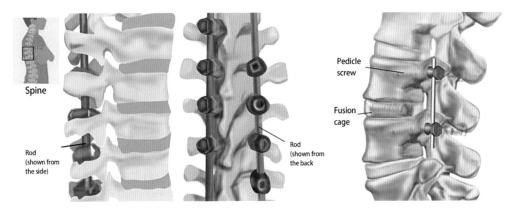

Figure 8.14   **Spinal fusion**

(4) Decompression

Chiari decompression

This is a procedure done for people who have a defect in the brain that controls balance.

This condition is also referred to as Arnold-Chiari malformation. Chiari decompression is the safest neurosurgery procedure for treating this condition. A bone at the back of the patient's skull is removed to improve their balance and coordination. **(Figure 8.15)**

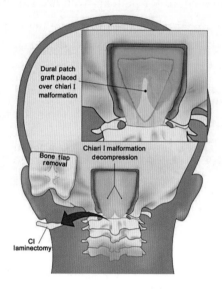

Figure 8.15 **Chiari decompression**

(5) Lumbar puncture

This is a simple procedure but a very effective one. Lumbar puncture is also known as spinal tap and is done to diagnose several underlying diseases affecting a patient's central nervous system. **(Figure 8.16)**

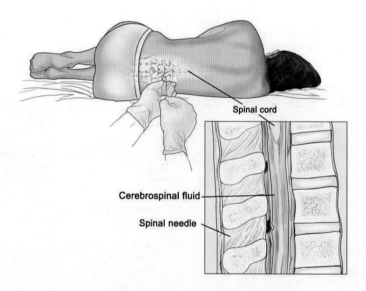

Figure 8.16 **Lumbar puncture**

(6) Lumbar drain (Figure 8.17)

- Prior to placement,complete a neuro assessment and vitals
- Position patient in decubitus (knee to chest) position or seated on the side of the bed leaning on a bedside table
- Blood present indicates a traumatic tap
- Apply an absorbent occlusive dressing that is assessed at least every 8 hours

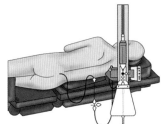

Figure 8.17 Lumbar drain

3. Endovascular procedures

(1) Carotid endarterectomy (Figure 8.18)

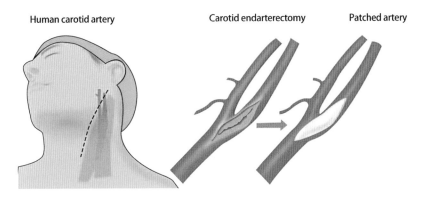

Figure 8.18 Carotid endarterectomy

(2) Coil embolization (Figure 8.19)

Endovascular(meaning within the blood vessel) embolization,or coiling,uses the natural access to the brain through the bloodstream via arteries to diagnosis and treat brain aneurysms. The goal of the treatment is to safely seal off the aneurysm and stop further blood from entering into the aneurysm and increasing the risk of rupture or possibly rebleeding.

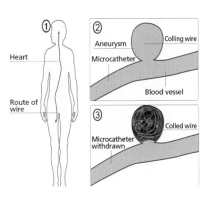

Figure 8.19 Coil embolization

(3) Femoral arterial puncture (Figure 8.20)

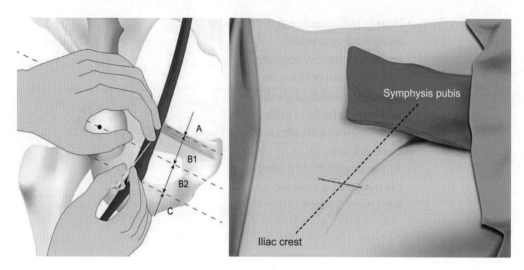

Figure 8.20 Femoral arterial puncture

4. Peripheral nerve surgery

(1) Carpel tunnel release

Carpal tunnel syndrome, diagnosed by clinical and electrodiagnostic studies. A fair trial of conservative management (behavior modification, splinting, etc.) is attempted first. Preoperatively, reassure patients that they will experience paresthesias during the recovery period, sometimes for a few weeks. This is part of the normal healing process; patients will often be distressed by paresthesias if not forewarned. (Figure 8.21)

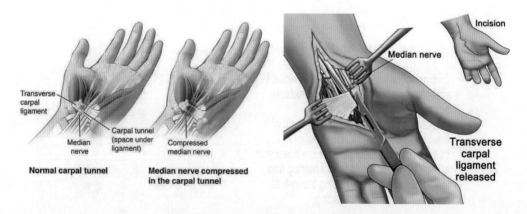

Figure 8.21 Carpel tunnel release

Technique:

➤ The incision is injected with local anesthetic (four parts lidocaine 0.5% with epinephrine, four parts bupivacaine 0.25%, one part sodium bicarbonate); some practitioners discourage the use of epinephrine in hand surgery; no tourniquet is necessary.

➤ Incise the skin with a No.15 blade and place a self retaining retractor. Deeper dissection will reveal the palmar fascia; incise this next and place the retractor deeper to keep the subcutaneous fat out of the way; bipolar may be used to shrink some of the more problematic fat away.

➤ Incise the distal portion of the flexor retinaculum with a No.15 blade until the median nerve is seen; use Metzenbaum scissors to divide the ligament proximally and distally completely.

➤ Have the assistant elevate the skin with a Senn retractor so that all bands of constrictive tissue, including fascia, may be divided for at least 3 to 4 cm proximally and 2 to 3 cm distally beyond the confines of the incision (for a total of 7 to 9 cm of nerve decompression).

➤ Irrigate, obtain hemostasis and close with 5–0 nylon vertical mattress sutures.

(2) Ulnar nerve release

Ulnar neuropathy is usually diagnosed by clinical examination and electrodiagnostic studies. A fair trial of conservative management (behavior modification, elbow padding, etc.) is attempted first. There are five points of entrapment of the ulnar nerve that must be released in this region (**Figure 8.22**):

➤ **The triceps fascia (arcade of Struthers)**

➤ **Medial intermuscular septum**

➤ **Ulnar groove**

➤ **The heads of the flexor carpi ulnaris (Osborne's ligament)**

➤ **The flexor-pronator aponeurosis**.

As in carpal tunnel syndrome, aggressive pursuit of nerve decompression beyond the confines of the incision eliminates points of entrapment that could limit nerve recovery.

Technique:

The incision is injected with local anesthetic (four parts lidocaine 0.5% with epinephrine, four parts bupivacaine 0.25%, one part sodium bicarbonate); no tourniquet is necessary.

Incise the skin with a No. 15 blade and place a self retaining retractor.

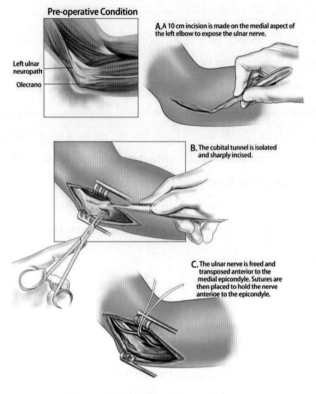

Pre-operative Condition

Left ulnar neuropath

Olecrano

A. A 10 cm incision is made on the medial aspect of the left elbow to expose the ulnar nerve.

B. The cubital tunnel is isolated and sharply incised.

C. The ulnar nerve is freed and transposed anterior to the medial epicondyle. Sutures are then placed to hold the nerve anterioe to the epicondyle.

Figure 8.22 Ulnar Nerve Release

Incise all connective tissue overlying the ulnar nerve within the incision; do not perform circumferential external neurolysis; do not manipulate the nerve if at all possible.

Have the assistant elevate the skin with a Senn retractor so that all bands of constrictive tissue, including fascia, may be divided for at least 4 cm more proximally than the most proximal extent of the incision; excise any portions of the medial intermuscular septum that may be compressing the nerve during this process.

Have the assistant elevate the skin with a Senn retractor so that all bands of constrictive tissue and fascia are divided for at least 4 cm distally to the distal-most extent of the incision. The fascia overlying the heads of the flexor carpi ulnaris that splits the heads of this muscle will be divided.

Irrigate the wound and close with 3–0 Vicryl suture and steri-strips.

(3) Tracheostomy

Tracheostomy can be performed in theatres (open surgical tracheostomy) or at the bedside (percutaneous dilatation tracheostomy), the latter being common in intensive care unit (ICU). **(Figure 8.23)**

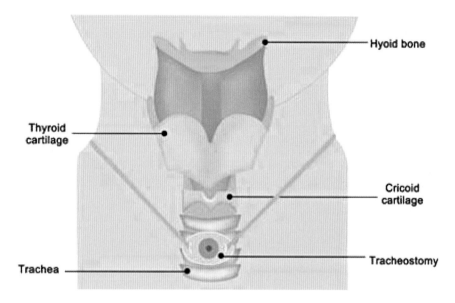

Figure 8.23 **Tracheostomy**

Surgical tracheostomy:

➢ The patient is supine with head extension and under general anesthesia.

➢ The incision is 2-3cm from the second tracheal ring down.

➢ Divide the thyroid isthmus if needed.

➢ Make a hole between the third and fourth tracheal rings, removing the anterior portion of the tracheal ring.

➢ The tracheostomy tube is inserted.

Percutaneous tracheostomy:

➢ Percutaneous placement of a tracheostomy is performed using guidewires and dilators.

➢ Guidewire is placed between the first and second tracheal rings.

➢ Gradually, the hole size is increased using dilators of varying sizes passed over the guidewire.

8.7.2 Basic Neurosurgical Approaches

Anterior fossa:

➢ Pterional approach

➢ Frontal and bifrontal approach

➢ Orbitozygomatic approach

➢ Anterior Interhemispheric approach

Middle fossa:

Temporal approach

Sub temporal approach

Combined anterior and posterior petrosectomy

Posterior fossa:

Translabyrinthine approach

Presigmoid

Retrosigmoid

Lateral suboccipital

Far lateral and extreme lateral approach

Midline suboccipital infratentorial approach

8.7.3 Basic Investigations in Neurosurgery

Brain scans include several imaging techniques used to diagnose tumors, blood vessel malformations, stroke, injuries, abnormal brain development, and bleeding in the brain. Types of brain scans include computed tomography (CT), magnetic resonance imaging (MRI), positron emission tomography (PET), and single proton emission (SPECT) scans. **(Figure 8.24)**

B	Blood	Blood
C	Can	Cisterns
B	Be	Brain
V	Very	Ventricles
B	Bad	Bone

Figure 8.24 **Mnemonic for interpreting CT head scan**

1. CT scan

A useful **mnemonic** that is used to read an emergency head CT scan is:

Blood Can Be Very Bad

Using a systematic approach will help to ensure that significant neuropathology will not be missed.

B: blood

Look for epidural hematoma, subdural hematoma, intraparenchymal hemorrhage, intraventricular hemorrhage, subarachnoid hemorrhage and (also) extracranial hemorrhage.

C: cisterns

Look for the presence of blood, effacement and asymmetry in four key cisterns (perimesencephalic, suprasellar, quadrigeminal and Sylvian cisterns).

B: brain

Look for asymmetry or effacement of the sulcal pattern, gray-white matter differentiation (including the insular ribbon sign), structural shifts and abnormal hypodensities (e.g., air, edema, fat) or hyperdensities (e.g., blood, calcification).

V: ventricles

Look for intraventricular hemorrhage, ventricular effacement or shift and hydrocephalus.

B: bone

Look for skull fractures (especially basal) on bone windows (soft tissue swelling, mastoid air cells, and paranasal sinuses fluid in the setting of trauma should raise the possibility of a skull fracture; intracranial air means that the skull and the dura have been violated somewhere).

CT vs. MRI: What to order?	
CT	**MRI**
Acute neurological events:	**Acute (susally after CT):**
-Stroke	-Stroke
-Trauma	-Encephalitis
-Worst HA of life	
-Acute mental status change	**Subacute and chronic:**
-First seizure	-Progressive, subacute, or chronic neurological deficit
-Neurosurgery immediate post-op	-TIAs, h/o of stroke
	-Brain tumors
Follow up	-Metastatic disease
-Acute infarcts	-Dementia
-Hemorrhage	Epilepsy
-Hydrocephaius	-Chronic headaches
	-MS
	-Developmental delay
	-Pituitary disorders
	-Cranial nerve dysfunction

2. MR images and sequences

Many factors lead to the production of the final MR image. Different combinations of these will be useful for different clinical presentations, but here are some examples of common images sequences:

a. T_1 weighted and T_2 weighted imaging (T_1WI and T_2WI)

b. DWI and ADC

c. FLAIR

d. STIR

(1) T_1 and T_2 weighted images (Figure 8.25)

- **T_1 — ONE** tissue is bright: **fat.**

   T_2 — TWO tissues are bright: **fat and water (WW2 — water is white in T_2).**

- T_1 is the most "anatomical" image, conversely, the cerebrospinal fluid (CSF) is bright in T_2 due to its' water content.

- T_2 is generally the more commonly used, but T_1 can be used as a reference for anatomical structures or to distinguish between fat versus bright signals.

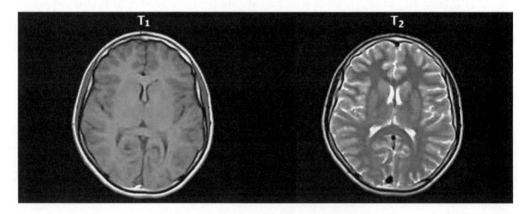

Figure 8.25 T_1 and T_2 weighted images

Additional feature of T_1 and T_2 weighted images:

1) **Fat suppressed:** the fat can be suppressed to enable a better view of pathology in and around anatomical structures , particularly edema. This is useful in adrenal tumors or bone marrow pathology, where the image will appear homogeneous with surrounding tissue due to fat content.

2) **Gadolinium enhanced:** gadolinium enhances vasculature (that is, arteries) or pathologically vascular tissues (examples: intracranial metastases, meningiomas). This process involves injecting 5-15ml of contrast intravenously, with images taken shortly

after that. Gadolinium appears bright in signal, allowing for detection of detailed abnormalities (example: intracranial pathologies). Typical intracranial abscesses have a "ring-enhancement" pattern, while metastases enhance homogeneously.

Meningioma will have a homogeneous enhancement after the contrast and a "dural tail," meaning the lesion appears continuous with the dura. **(Figure 8.26)**

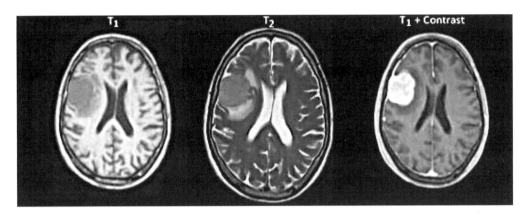

Figure 8.26 **Meningioma is shown more clearly by gadolinium contrast with a dural tail**

(2) Inversion recovery (IR) sequences: these types of images are manipulations of T_1 and T_2. They nullify certain tissue types based on their inversion timings, thereby stopping tissues such as fat and CSF from appearing as bright signals. This is helpful to identify pathological signals. The two types are discussed below.

> **Short tau inversion recovery (STIR):** STIR is based on a T_2 image, but the image is manipulated to nullify fat (and any other materials with similar signals). Unlike fat-suppressed images, however, STIR can not be used with gadolinium contrast. **(Figure 8.27)**

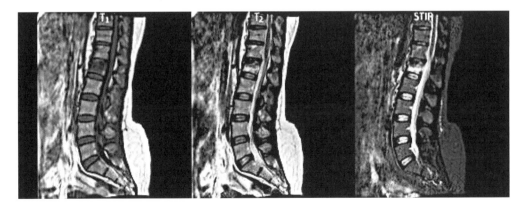

Figure 8.27 **STIR highlighting marrow oedema in L$_1$ vertebra, indicative of a fracture**

> **Fluid attenuated inversion recovery (FLAIR):** FLAIR is similar to T_2; however, the CSF signal is nullified. This is particularly useful for evaluating structures in the central nervous system (CNS), including the periventricular areas, sulci, and gyri. For example, FLAIR can be used to identify plaques in multiple sclerosis, subtle edema after a stroke, and pathology in other conditions whereby CSF may interfere with interpretations. **(Figure 8.28)**

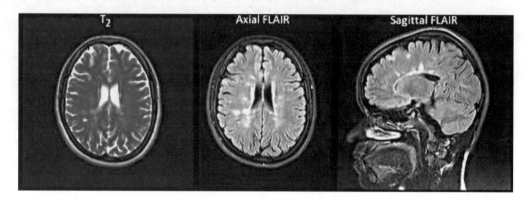

Figure 8.28 **Multiple sclerotic plaques in periventricular regions and corpus collosum**

(3) Diffused weighted imaging (DWI): DWI is an imaging modality that combines T_2 images with the diffusion of water. With DWI scans, ischemia can be visualized within minutes of occurring. This is because DWI has a high sensitivity for water diffusion, thereby detecting the physiological changes immediately after a stroke.

A systemic approach to MRI interpretation:

- Verify detail.
- Look at the T_2 weighted images.
- Compare different MRI image sequences (T_1, T_2, STIR, FLAIR, DWI).
- Compare against other image modalities (ultrasound, CT, plain film).
- Compare against previous images:

Consider the clinical context: finally, place your findings in context with the clinical presentation to ascertain a radiological diagnosis:

✓ Are the symptoms acute or chronic?

✓ How unwell is the patient?

✓ Does the imaged pathology correlates with the presenting symptoms?

Summary:

We have outlined the basics of different types of MRI, along with key examples. A lot has been covered, and a lot has not, but this will give you a good understanding of the fundamentals of MRI.

3. DSA technique

Digital subtraction angiography **(DSA)** is used to produce images of the blood vessels without interfering shadows from overlapping tissues. This provides a clear view of the vessels and allows for a lower dose of contrast medium.

Procedural technique:

For every purpose, there is at least one technique, but common to them all is the application of DSA for visualization **(Figure 8.29)**:

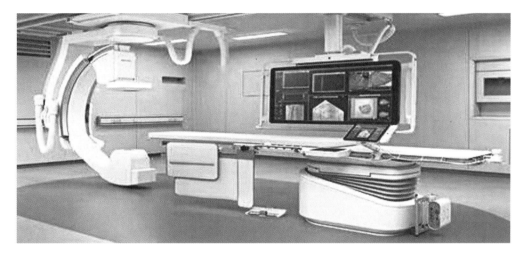

Figure 8.29 **Digital subtraction angiography (DSA)**

The patient lies on the angiography table.

Local anesthesia is administered at the intended puncture site (usually lidocaine hydrochloride 1% or 2% weight in volume)

In certain procedures (e.g., a child undergoing cerebral angiography), general anesthesia is performed.

The Seldinger technique is used to gain access to a blood vessel. A standard access kit includes a straight 18 gauge needle and .035" guidewires, on which the diagnostic and therapeutic catheters are threaded.

In many cases, a micro-introducer access kit (.018" guidewire threaded through a 21 gauge initial access needle) is used for access, either for the entire procedure or to be replaced with the standard kit. Using a micro-introducer facilitates less traumatic entry and can be retrieved without massive bleeding.

8.8 Major Abbreviations and Symbols

. Full stop or period

, Comma

: Colon

; Semicolon

? Question mark

( ) Round bracket

[ ]Square bracket

"" Quatation marks (double quotes)

A' Apostrophe

A... Ellipsis points

A! Exclamation mark

<u>A</u> Underline

A-B Hyphen

A/B Stroke or slash

* Asterix

Index

Appendix

No.	Medical terminology	IPA phonetic	Everyday term
1	Anterior	ænˈtɪərɪə	Front
2	Posterior	pɒsˈtɪərɪə	Back
3	Lateral	lætərəl	Side
4	Right lateral Left lateral	raɪt lætərəl lɛft lætərəl	Right side Left side
5	Dorsal	dɔːsəl	Upper side
6	Ventral	vɛntrəl	On or near the belly
7	Medial	miːdjəl	Toward the midline
8	Proximal	prɒksɪm (ə) l	Nearer to
9	Distal	dɪstəl	Farther from
10	Superior	sju (ː)ˈpɪərɪə	Above
11	Inferior	ɪnˈfɪərɪə	Below
12	Cephalic	kɛˈfælɪk	Toward the head
13	Caudal	kɔːdl	Toward the spine
14	Superficial (external)	sjuːpəˈfɪʃəl	Toward the surface
15	Deep (Internal)	diːp	Toward the center
16	Coronal Plane	kɒrənl pleɪn	Frontal plane
17	Sagittal	sædʒɪtl	Middle plane
18	Axial Plane	æksɪəl pleɪn	Horizontal plane
19	Prone	prəʊn	Face up
20	Supine	sjuːˈpaɪn	Face down
21	Cephalic	kɛˈfælɪk	Head
22	Frontal	frʌntl	Forehead
23	Ocular	ɒkjʊlə	Eyes
24	Oral	ɔːrəl	Mouth

continued

No.	Medical terminology	IPA phonetic	Everyday term
25	Nasal	neɪzəl	Nose
26	Mandibular	mænˈdɪbjʊlə	Lower jaw
27	Maxilla	mækˈsɪlə	Upper jaw
28	Cervical	sə(ː)ˈvaɪkəl	Neck
29	Mentum	mɛntəm	Chin
30	Laryngeal prominence	ləˈrɪndʒɪəlˈprɒmɪnəns	Adam's apple
31	Axilla	ækˈsɪlə	Armpit
32	Clavicle	klævɪkl	Collar bone
33	Mammary	mæməri	Breast
34	Sternum	stɜːnəm	Breast bone
35	Acromion	əˈkroʊmiən	Shoulder tip
36	Humerus	hjumərəs	Shoulder
37	Abdomen	æbdəmɛn	Belly, tummy
38	Umbilical	ʌmbɪˈlaɪkəl	Navel belly button
39	Brachial	ˈbreɪkɪəl	Arm
40	Antebrachial	anteˈbrakhium	Forearm
41	Thorax	θɔːræks	Chest
42	Antecubital fossa	anteˈbrakhium/ˈfɒsə	Crook of the elbow
43	Ulna	ʌlnə	Forearm
44	Carpal	kɑːpəl	Wrist
45	Palmar	ˈpælmə	Palm
46	Iliac	ˈɪlɪæk	Flank
47	Digits/Phalanges	ˈdɪdʒɪts/fæˈlændʒɪ	Fingers
48	Genitalia	dʒɛnəˈtɑljə	Genital
49	Femoral	ˈfɛmərəl	Thigh
50	Inguinal	ˈɪŋgwɪnl	Groin
51	Patella	pəˈtɛlə	Knee cap
52	Tibia	ˈtɪbɪə	Shin

continued

No.	Medical terminology	IPA phonetic	Everyday term
53	Talus	ˈteɪləs	Ankle
54	Dorsum pedis	ˈdorsum/ˈpeːdis	Upper part of the foot
55	Phalanges	fæˈlændʒɪz	Toes
56	Hallux	ˈhælaks	Big toe
57	Onycho	ˈonikəu	Toe nail
58	Plantar	ˈplæntə	Sole of the foot
59	Metatarsal	metəˈtaːsəl	Ball of the foot
60	Calcaneus	kælˈkeɪniəs	Heel
61	Parietal	pəˈraɪətəl	Crown of the head
62	Occipital	ɒkˈsɪpɪtl	Back of the head
63	Nuchal	ˈnjuːkl	Nape of the neck
64	Thoracic region	θɔːˈræsɪkˈriːdʒən	Upper back
65	Glenohumerus joint	Glenohumerus dʒɔɪnt	Shoulder joint
66	Scapula	ˈskæpjələ	Shoulder blade
67	Humerus	ˈhjumərəs	Upper arm
68	Olecranon	oʊˈlɛkrənan	Tip of the elbow
69	Vertebrae	ˈvɜːtɪbriː	Spine
70	Lumbar region	ˈlʌmbəˈriːdʒən	Lower back
71	Os coxae	ɒs coxae	Hip bone
72	Iliac region	ˈɪlɪækˈriːdʒən	Flank
73	Sacrum	ˈseɪkrəm	Sacrum
74	Gluteal	gluˈtiːəs	Buttock
75	Loss of Consciousness	lɒs əvˈkɒnʃəsnɪs	Passed out
76	Cerebral hemorrhage	ˈsɛrɪbrəlˈhɛmərɪdʒ	Bleeding in the brain
77	Vomiting	vɑmətɪŋ	Bringing up food
78	Indigestion	ɪndaɪˈdʒɛstʃən	Stomach problem
79	Pain	peɪn	Unpleasant feeling

continued

No.	Medical terminology	IPA phonetic	Everyday term
80	Deep vein thrombosis (DVT)	dip veɪn θrɑmˈboʊsəs (di-vi-ti)	Blood clot in one of the deep vein of the lower leg
81	Hypoglycemia	ˌhaɪpoʊglaɪˈsimiə	Abnormal low blood sugar
82	Malaise	mæˈleɪz	Feeling queasy/Uneasiness
83	Contusion	kənˈtjuːʒən	Bruise
84	Wound	wuːnd	A Sore
85	Diarrhea	ˌdaɪəˈriə	Running stomach/ Passing loose stool
86	Dysmenorrhea	dɪsmɛnəˈriə	Period pain/Menstrual pain
87	Conjunctivitis	kənˌdʒʌŋktɪˈvaɪtɪs	Red eye
88	Allergic rhinitis	əˈlɜːdʒɪk raɪˈnaɪtɪs	Hay fever
89	Rhinorrhea	ˌraɪnəˈriə	Runny nose
90	Dyspepsia	dɪsˈpɛpsɪə	Heart burn
91	Cystitis	sɪsˈtaɪtɪs	Bladder infection
92	Respiratory disease	rɪˈspɪrət (ə) ri dɪˈziːz	Breathing problems
93	Allergies	ælədʒiz	Sensitivities to medication or chemicals
94	Epilepsy	ɛpɪlɛpsi	Block –out or seizures
95	Asthma	æsmə	Wheezing
96	Urticaria	Urticaria	Itchiness
97	Nausea	ˈnɔːziə	Sick feeling
98	Hyperglycemia / Diabetes	haɪpərglaɪˈsimiə / ˌdaɪəˈbiːtiːz	High blood sugar
99	Pyrexia	Pyrexia	Fever
100	Bradycardia	ˌbrædəˈkardiə	Slow Pulse
101	Tachycardia	tækɪˈkaːdɪə	Fast Pulse
102	Hypotension	ˌhaɪpoʊˈtɛnʃən	Low blood pressure
103	Hypertension	ˌhaɪpərˈtɛnʃən	High blood pressure
104	Thrombosis	θrɑmˈboʊsəs	Blood clot
105	Agoraphobia	əˌɡɔrəˈfoʊbiə	Fear of being in a public place
106	Aphasia	əˈfeɪʒə	Loss or defect in speech communication

continued

No.	Medical terminology	IPA phonetic	Everyday term
107	Astrocytoma	æstrəʊsaɪˈtəʊmə	A neuroglia *(neu/ro/glia)* tumor composed of astrocytes *(as/tro/cytes)*
108	Coprolalia	koːproːlaːˈli	Compulsive use of obscene words
109	Corticospinal	Corticospinal	Pertaining to the cerebral *(ce/re/bral)* cortex and spinal cord
110	Decerebrate	dɪˈsɛrəbrət	Having no cerebral function
111	Dementia	dɪˈmɛnʃɪə	Irreversible loss of intellectual function
112	Dyslexia	dɪsˈlɛksɪə	Difficulty in reading
113	Encephalitis	ɛnkɛfəˈlaɪtɪs	Inflammation *(in/fla/ma/tion)* of the brain
114	Encephalomalacia	ɛnˌsɛfəloʊməˈleɪʃə,-ʃɪə	Softening of brain tissue
115	Epilepsy	ɛpɪlɛpsi	A chronic disease involving periodic sudden bursts of electric activity from brain resulting in seizure
116	Ganglionectomy	gæŋglɪəˈnɛktəmi	Surgical removal of a ganglion
117	Glioma	glaɪˈəumə	A neuroglia tumor
118	Hallucination	həˌlusəˈneɪʃən	A false perception unrelated to reality or external stimulus
119	Hemiparesis	ˌhɛmipəˈrɪsɪs	Partial paralysis *(pa/ra/ly/sis)* of one side of the body
120	Hemiplegia	ˌhɛməˈplidʒɪə	Paralysis of one side of the body
121	Heterophasia	hɛtrˌəfejʒə	Uttering words that are different from those intended
122	Hydrocephalus	ˌhaɪdrəˈsɛfələs	Increased accumulation of cerebrospinal *(ce/re/bro/spi/nal)* fluid (CSF) in or around the brain as a result of obstruction to flow
123	Insomnia	ɪnˈsɒmnɪə	Insufficient or non-restorative sleep despite ample opportunity to sleep
124	Intracerebellar	ɪntraˌsɛrəˈbɛlə	Within the cerebellum *(se/re/bel/lum)*
125	Medullary	mɛˈdʌləri	Pertaining to the medulla *(me/dul/la)*
126	Megalomania	mɛgələʊˈmeɪnɪə	Exaggerated self-importance, delusion of grandeur

continued

No.	Medical terminology	IPA phonetic	Everyday term
127	Meningioma	məˌnɪndʒiˈoʊmə	Tumor of the meninges
128	Meningitis	mɛnɪnˈdʒaɪtɪ	Inflammation of the meninges
129	Meningocele	menĩŋgoˈsele	Hernia of the meninges through the skull or spinal column
130	Myelodysplasia	myelodis-ˈplā-zh(ē-)ə	Abnormal development of the spinal cord
131	Narcolepsy	ˈnɑrkəˌlɛpsi	Condition marked by sudden episode of sleep
132	Narcosis	narˈkoʊsɪs	State of stupor
133	Neurilemoma/ Schwannoma	neurolə-ˈmō-mə/ eʃbaˈnoma	A tumor of the sheath of peripheral *(pe/rif/er/al)* nerve
134	Neurotoxic	ˌnʊəroʊˈtɒksɪk	Harmful or poisonous nerve or neuron tissue
135	Paralysis	pəˈræləsəs	Temporary or permanent loss of function
136	Parkinsonism	ˈpɑrkɪnsəˌnɪzɪm	A disorder originating in the basal ganglia and characterized by slow movement, tremor, rigidity, and masklike face
137	Psychosomatic	saɪˌkoʊsəˈmætɪk	Pertaining to the mind and body (soma)
138	Radiculopathy	ræˈdɪkjʊləʊpəθɪ	Any disease of the spinal nerve root
139	Seizure	siːʒə	A sudden attack as in epilepsy
140	Shingles	ʃɪŋglz	An acute viral infection that follows nerve pathways causing small lesion on the skin
141	Somnolence	sɒmnələns	Sleepiness
142	Supra-ventricular	sjuːprəvɛnˈtrɪkjʊlə	Above a ventricle
143	Tetraplegia / Quadriplegia	tetraplegia /quadriplegia	Paralysis of all four limbs
144	Thalamotomy	θælamowtəmi	Incision of the thalamus

Useful References

[1] VIRGINIA A. English for medical purposes: doctors. Lulu publishing services, 2012.

[2] HAL B. Neuroanatomy through clinical cases. 2nd ed. Sunderland: Sinauer Associate Inc, 2010.

[3] GERIANT F. Neurological examination made easy. 5th ed. New York: Churchill Livingstone, Elservier, 2013.

[4] GLENDINNING E H, HOWARD R. Professional English in use medicine. Cambridge: Cambridge University Press, 2006.

[5] MELODIE H. Medical English clear & simple: a practice-based approach to English for ESL healthcare professionals. , Philadelphia: F.A. Davis Company, 2010.

[6] LINARES O, DALY D T, DALY G A. Plain English for doctors and other medical scientists. New York: Oxford University Press Inc., 2017.

[7] SAM M C. Oxford English for careers. New York: Oxford University Press, 2010.

[8] Tips for writing better science papers: education[2021-11-01]. https://www.chemistryviews.org/details/education/5202161/Tips_for_Writing_Better_Science_Papers.html.

[9] Writing a medical case study[2021-11-01]. https://www.prrm.pl/?p=49678299.

[10] WALLWORK W, SOUTHERN A. 100 tips to avoid mistakes in academic writing and presenting[2021-11-01]. https://dokumen.pub/100-tips-to-avoid-mistakes-in-academic-writing-and-presenting-1st-edition-3030442136-9783030442132-9783030442149.html.

图书在版编目（CIP）数据

神经外科住院医师规范化培训实用英语 / 王向宇，
（利比）奥古斯丁·K. 巴拉（Augustine K. Ballah）主编
. —北京：人民卫生出版社，2022.6
　ISBN 978–7–117–32926–2

　Ⅰ.①神…　Ⅱ.①王…②奥…　Ⅲ.①神经外科学 –
英语　Ⅳ.①R651

　中国版本图书馆 CIP 数据核字（2022）第 043162 号

人卫智网	www.ipmph.com	医学教育、学术、考试、健康， 购书智慧智能综合服务平台
人卫官网	www.pmph.com	人卫官方资讯发布平台

神经外科住院医师规范化培训实用英语
Shenjing Waike Zhuyuan Yishi Guifanhua Peixun Shiyong Yingyu

主　　编：王向宇［利比里亚］Augustine K. Ballah
出版发行：人民卫生出版社（中继线 010-59780011）
地　　址：北京市朝阳区潘家园南里 19 号
邮　　编：100021
E - mail：pmph @ pmph.com
购书热线：010-59787592　010-59787584　010-65264830
印　　刷：北京顶佳世纪印刷有限公司
经　　销：新华书店
开　　本：787×1092　1/16　印张：10
字　　数：207 千字
版　　次：2022 年 6 月第 1 版
印　　次：2022 年 9 月第 1 次印刷
标准书号：ISBN 978-7-117-32926-2
定　　价：79.00 元
打击盗版举报电话：010-59787491　E-mail：WQ @ pmph.com
质量问题联系电话：010-59787234　E-mail：zhiliang @ pmph.com
数字融合服务电话：4001118166　　E-mail：zengzhi @ pmph.com

55检